MAGNETIC RESONANCE IMAGING
OF CARCINOMA OF THE URINARY BLADDER

SERIES IN RADIOLOGY

VOLUME 21

The titles published in this series are listed at the end of this volume.

MAGNETIC RESONANCE IMAGING OF CARCINOMA OF THE URINARY BLADDER

JELLE O. BARENTSZ

Department of Radiodiagnostics, University of Nijmegen,
St. Radboud Hospital, Nijmegen, The Netherlands

FRANS M. J. DEBRUYNE

Department of Urology, University of Nijmegen,
St. Radboud Hospital, Nijmegen, The Netherlands

and

SJEF H. J. RUIJS

Department of Radiodiagnostics, University of Nijmegen,
St. Radboud Hospital, Nijmegen, The Netherlands

Preface by

H. Hricak

Professor of Radiology and Urology, UCSF, U.S.A.

and

R. Hohenfellner

Professor of Urology, Mainz, F.R.G.

KLUWER ACADEMIC PUBLISHERS

DORDRECHT / BOSTON / LONDON

Library of Congress Cataloging in Publication Data

Barentsz, Jelle O.
    [Kernspin tomografie bij het urineblaascarcinoom. English]
    Magnetic resonance imaging of carcinoma of the urinary bladder /
Jelle O. Barentsz, Frans M.J. Debruyne, Sjef H.J. Ruijs.
        p.   cm. -- (Series in radiology ; 21)
    Translation of: Kernspin tomographie bij het urineblaascarcinoom.
    Includes bibliographical references.

    1. Bladder--Cancer--Magnetic resonance imaging.   I. Debruyne, F.
M. J., 1941-   . II. Ruijs, Sjef, H. J.   III. Title.   IV. Series.
    [DNLM: 1. Bladder Neoplasms--diagnosis.   2. Magnetic Resonance
Imaging.   W1 SE719 v. 21 / WJ 504 B248k]
    RC280.B5B3513 1990
    616.99'46207548--dc20
DNLM/DLC
for Library of Congress   90-4894

ISBN-13: 978-94-010-6778-2   e-ISBN-13: 978-94-009-0651-8
DOI: 10.1007/978-94-009-0651-8

Published by Kluwer Academic Publishers,
P.O. Box 17, 3300 AA Dordrecht, The Netherlands.

Kluwer Academic Publishers incorporates
the publishing programmes of
D. Reidel, Martinus Nijhoff, Dr W. Junk and MTP Press.

Sold and distributed in the U.S.A. and Canada
by Kluwer Academic Publishers,
101 Philip Drive, Norwell, MA 02061, U.S.A.

In all other countries, sold and distributed
by Kluwer Academic Publishers Group,
P.O. Box 322, 3300 AH Dordrecht, The Netherlands.

Printed on acid-free paper

CONTENTS

PREFACE by H. Hricak		VIII
PREFACE by R. Hohenfellner		IX
ACKNOWLEDGMENTS		XI

I.   **INTRODUCTION**

1.1	**Magnetic spin tomography**	2
1.2	**Carcinoma of the urinary bladder**	3
1.2.1	General aspects	3
1.2.2	Method of clinical staging	5
1.3	**Diagnostic imaging of carcinoma of the urinary bladder**	6
1.3.1	Intravenous urography	6
1.3.2	Ultrasound	7
1.3.3	Computed Tomography	8
1.3.4	Lymphography	8
1.3.5	Magnetic Resonance Imaging	10
1.4	**Aims and design of this study**	10

II.   **GENERAL PRINCIPLES OF MRI**

2.1	**Introduction**	14
2.2	**Basic physics of MRI**	14
2.2.1	Nuclear spins, resonant frequency	14
2.2.2	Spin imaging: proton density, T_1 and T_2 relaxation times	15
2.3	**Image contrast**	18
2.3.1	'Inherent' tissue contrast, image contrast	18
2.3.2	Adjustable factors, pulse sequences	19
2.3.2.1	*Spin-echo pulse sequence*	19
2.3.2.2	*Inversion recovery pulse sequence*	20
2.3.2.3	*Pulse sequence optimization*	21
2.4	**Strength of the magnetic field**	21
2.5	**Artifacts**	21
2.5.1	Aliasing (wraparound) artifact	22
2.5.2	Fat-shift artifact	22
2.5.3	Artifacts caused by patients' movement	22
2.5.4	Metal artifacts	23
2.6	**Advantages of MRI over other imaging techniques**	23
2.7	**Disadvantages of MRI compared with other imaging techniques**	24
2.8	**Safety of MRI**	25
2.8.1	Short term effects	25
2.8.1.1	*Static magnetic field*	25

8.1.2	*Effects of electrical currents induced by the main magnetic field varying in time*	26
2.8.1.3	*Warming/heating effects of RF signals*	26
2.8.2	Long-term effects	26
2.9	**Contraindications for MRI investigation**	27

III. TECHNICAL ASPECTS OF MRI SPECIFICIALLY RELEVANT TO PATIENTS WITH URINARY BLADDER CARCINOMA

3.1	**Introduction, optimal conditions for examination**	30
3.2	**Patient-related factors**	30
3.2.1	Voluntary motion artifacts	30
3.2.2	Involuntary motion artifacts	30
3.2.3	Bladder distension	30
3.3	**Pulse sequence optimization**	30
3.3.1	Literature review	31
3.3.2	Evaluation of sequences most frequently used in the literature	33
3.3.2.1	*T_1-weighted sequences*	33
3.3.2.2	*T_2-weighted sequences*	34
3.3.2.3	*Proton-weighted sequences*	37
3.3.3	Determination of the optimal pulse sequence (1.5 T)	37
3.3.3.1	*T_1 and T_2 calculations to optimize the pulse sequence*	38
3.3.3.2	*Pulse sequence optimization by means of 'contrast matrices'*	39
3.3.3.3	*Pulse sequence optimization by means of 'synthetic imaging'*	40
3.3.4	Interim conclusion	43
3.4	**Body-coil MRI versus (double) surface-coil MRI**	43
3.4.1	Results at a field strength of 0.5 T	48
3.4.1.1	*Patients and methods*	48
3.4.1.2	*Results*	50
3.4.1.3	*Discussion*	51
3.4.2	Results at a field strength of 1.5 T	52
3.4.2.1	*Patients and methods*	52
3.4.2.2	*Results*	54
3.4.2.3	*Discussion*	54
3.4.3	Interim conclusion	54
3.5	**Comparison of staging results at 0.5 T and 1.5 T**	55
3.5.1	Introduction	55
3.5.2	Patients, methods, and results	55
3.5.3	Discussion	58
3.6	**Conclusion and protocol to be followed**	58

IV.   NORMAL MR IMAGES:
CORRELATION WITH KNOWN ANATOMIC PROPORTIONS

4.1   **Normal MR images of the pelvis**   60

4.1.1   The male pelvis   60

4.1.2   The female pelvis   64

4.2   **Correlation of MR images with anatomic sections**   66

4.3   **Correlations of MR images with sections of resected specimens**   74

V.   STAGING OF CARCINOMA OF THE URINARY BLADDER ON THE
BASIS OF MRI RESULTS

5.1   **Introduction**   80

5.1.1   Survey of groups of patient   80

5.2   **Evaluation of MRI, CT, and the clinical staging method compared with postoperative**
        histopathologic staging based on cystectomy and autopsy specimens   81

5.2.1   Patients and methods   81

5.2.2   Results   82

5.2.2.1 *Patients*   82

5.2.2.2 *MR images of resected specimens*   88

5.2.3   Discussion   91

5.2.4   Interim conclusion   92

5.3.   **Evaluation of staging with MRI and CT by using a combination of clinical staging and**
        follow-up as a reference   92

5.3.1   Patients and methods   93

5.3.2   Results   94

5.3.3   Discussion   96

5.3.4   Interim conclusion   100

5.4   **Evaluation of staging with MRI by using a combination of clinical staging and follow-up**
        as a reference   100

5.4.1   Patients, methods, and results   101

5.4.2   Discussion   101

5.4.3. Interim conclusion   101

VI.   DISCUSSION, CONCLUSIONS AND FUTURE PERSPECTIVES

6.1   **Discussion and conclusions**   104

6.2   **Future prospects**   107

6.2.1   Surface coils   107

6.2.2   Contrast agents   107

6.2.3   Fast sequences   108

VII. SUMMARY   112

REFERENCES   116

PREFACE

Carcinoma of the urinary bladder is a common (in the USA it is the fifth most common form of cancer in males and tenth most common form of cancer in females) malignancy and one in which noninvasive staging by imaging plays such an important role.

This book presents a complete approach to MR imaging of carcinoma of the urinary bladder from a detailed discussion of the value of MRI in the diagnosis of the urinary bladder to the history of the procedure.

The technical discussion of the general principles of MRI including the optimal pulse sequences to be used and factors that influence the quality of images are included in this book. The safety factors are also presented along with contraindications.

The application of a double surface coil with the field strength of 0.5T provides the fine quality of the illustrations. The atlas of comparative anatomy by MRI on normal volunteers and post-mortem specimens as well as MR images on patients with bladder tumors and post-surgery specimens is unique. The results of the clinical imaging studies in patients with carcinoma of the bladder, comparing the relative value of clinical staging, MR, CT and lymphography, are helpful in showing the advantages of MRI.

This book brings new information in clear, well illustrated form. The value of this work lies in providing rational recommendations on imaging based on comparison and methodical analysis of data. This book, with the excellent illustrations and basic information on such an important subject will be extremely helpful to oncologists, oncologic urologists and to radiologists facing these problems.

Meticulous research of this type will further advance the treatment of cancer through noninvasive staging by imaging.

Hedvig Hricak, M.D.

Professor of Radiology and Urology
University of California, San Francisco.

PREFACE

Within a time-period of only 10 years the Department of Urology, under the direction of Frans Debruyne, developed into one of today's most important European urology departments of high international standard.

All the more there was eager expectation for the response to the following publication, which is dedicated to a new imaging system. At a time when the costs of more and more extensive diagnostic procedures are developing contrarily to stagnant therapeutic concepts, even the title of such a book is a challenge. All of us still have in mind the lectures on the advantages of intravesical ultrasound diagnostics filling the congress halls, and just after a long time of experience the benefit of this method turned out to be doubtful.

Is it possible to improve the so far disappointing results of computer diagnostics for the preoperative staging of bladder carcinomas to that extent that is will be effective enough to allow for a therapeutic decision?
Does MRI enable documentation of the response-kinetics which is an important parameter in chemo- and radiotherapy in the temporal course of tumor formation?
Is the MRI superior to CT and ultrasound concerning sensitivity and specification?

If so, a series of secured indications in the urological field, as e.g. the investigation of obscure neurogenic micturition disturbances or the differential diagnosis of masses in the small pelvis, just to mention a few of them, would be extended by another very important one.

But, to tell you at once, as expected – this book offers much more!

The reader should not fall into the usual trend and start the studies from the end. Only if you read the whole book with the same accuracy with which it had been written you will be able to device the expected benefit from it.
We address our full approval to the author and the publishing house for the work accomplished with much effort and last but not least for the extremely successful design.
The long-lasting relationship between radiologists and urologists has not always been free of disputes. From both sides there were discussions concerning the overlapping fields of radiodiagnostics.

Isotope diagnostics, computer tomography and now MRI brought the two faculties more closely together – for the benefit of the patient – a fact which has to pointed out as a very important aspect of this book.

R. Hohenfellner, M.D.

Professor of Urology
Klinikum der Johannes
Gutenberg-Universität
Mainz, B.R.D.

ACKNOWLEDGMENTS

The investigation that forms the basis of this study was performed in the Department of Radiodiagnostics at St. Radboud Hospital in Nijmegen, in the MR Application Department of Philips Medical Systems Division in Best, and in the MRI Department of the University Hospital in Utrecht.

I would like to take this opportunity to thank Prof. Dr. G. Rosenbusch for his expert guidance throughout this study. I am grateful to Dr. J. A. M. Lemmens and Dr. H. F. M. Karthaus for their critical supervision of the section dealing with general magnetic resonance imaging and the clinical part of this book, respectively. Many thanks are due to Dr. Ir. L. J. T. O. van Erning for his help with the section on principles involved in magnetic resonance imaging.

I thank the Stichting Radiologisch Onderzoek Nijmegen and the following companies for their financial support: Siemens Nederland N.V., Kodak Nederland B.V., Terumo, Rooster Medical, Schering Nederland B.V., Nycomed B.V., Bard Nederland B.V., and Cook Europe B.V. Some of the MR images were printed by using Kodak's Laser Imager. Thanks to Siemens, it was possible to optimize the print quality of the hard copies of the MR images. The MR contrastmaterial that was used was supplied by Schering (Magnevist®).

Finally I would like to thank Mrs. B. Vollers-King for the translation of this book and Mrs. K. Spiller for the final corrections.

Permission granted from the Williams & Wilkins Co. (publishers of AJR) to publish parts of the contents and figures of section 3.4.1.

J.O. Barentsz, M.D., Ph.D.

I

INTRODUCTION

1.1 Magnetic spin tomography

The interaction between science and the development of new technology is very seen in the development of nuclear magnetic resonance (NMR) studies in medical diagnostics and research. During the past few years, NMR investigation has developed very rapidly in the field of medicine, and it promises to become one of the most valuable and multifaceted techniques for medical research.

The foundation of NMR was laid in 1924. In that year, Pauli discovered the existence of *nuclear magnetism* when he was looking for a reason for the structure of atomic spectra.[151] During the subsequent 15 years, various methods were developed to measure the magnetic properties of nuclei. This resulted in an exact description of the principle of NMR by Bloch et al.[22] in 1946. They described current induction in a 'receiver coil' as the result of exposing certain atoms to a homogeneous, strong magnetic field under the influence of another, alternating magnetic field at right angles to it. The frequency of the latter field had to be approximately the same as the resonant frequency of these atoms (see Chapter 2). During the same period, Purcell et al.[180] described the resonance absorption of nuclear magnetic moments in paraffin. Both investigators were able to determine the structure and diffusion properties of molecules with the help of these resonance absorption techniques. They were awarded the Nobel Prize in 1952 for their work.

Within 5 years, it was discovered that the electronic structure and movements of molecules could be studied easily by using NMR. Before long, NMR was being applied to many areas of physics and chemistry. Its sensitivity increased dramatically with the introduction of and improvement in computers and with the development of superconducting magnets with a very strong and homogeneous magnetic field. This made it feasible to perform reliable investigations of the composition and properties of small amounts of biochemical material and solutions of macromolecules. Some observations were made on biological tissues: in 1971, Damadian[50] reported differences in nuclear magnetism (relaxation times) between tumor and normal tissue of rats. The idea also began to emerge that the inhomogeneity of magnetic fields could be used to determine the spatial arrangement of nuclei. Analogous to the digital construc-

tion of the image in computed tomography (CT), in 1973, Lauterbur[137] described the possibility of producing images of cross sections of objects by using NMR. The practical application of this was supported by the Cooley-Tukey fast Fourier transform algorithm (introduced in 1965). With this Fourier transformation, it became possible, under the influence of a magnetic-field gradient, to reconstruct an image on the monitor via a computer calculation.[69]

When the medical world realized the potential use of NMR, ideas, techniques, and equipment that had been developed during the previous 25 years were basically already available. This promoted considerably the growth of this branch of technology and its application to medical problems. Many concepts now generally used by medical researchers working in the field of NMR were discovered and defined during the starting phase, before any medical application for NMR was known. The influence of 'paramagnetic substances' was described by Bloch et al.[22] as early as 1946. Nowadays, paramagnetic substances are commonly used in NMR imaging. Relaxation times were studied by Bloch in 1946.[23] The properties and underlying theory of spin-echo signals were described by Hahn in 1950.[88] The spin-echo pulse sequence (see section 2.3.2.1) is now the most frequently used NMR sequence. The use of chemical-shift imaging is fairly new; however, the dependence of resonant frequency on certain tissue types has been known since 1949.[125, 178]

In spite of the fact that the conditions for applying NMR spectroscopy were present from an early stage, it was 1971 before the first description of its application to human tissue was published.[50] One supposed that, on the basis of T_1 and T_2 relaxation times, spin-echo NMR measurements could be used to differentiate between malignant and benign tissues. During subsequent years, the possibility of distinguishing malignant from benign tissues by means of NMR imaging was investigated further. The investigations were mainly aimed at the difference in T_1 and T_2 relaxation times. This was all related to *in vitro* experiments. The first NMR investigations *in vivo* were performed in 1972 on an experimental animal. No adverse effects were observed.[226]

In 1973, a method for creating images was described for the first time,[137] and this heralded the start of magnetic resonance imaging (MRI). The first NMR images were described in 1977. Mansfield and Maudsley[148] managed, with the help of a small magnet, to obtain an image of a finger. It proved possible to differentiate between fat, bone marrow, cortical bone, and tendons and to obtain images of blood circulation in the veins and arteries.[104] In 1979, Bottomley et al.[27] first demonstrated images of a hepatoma in the liver of a live rat. It was apparently possible, by using MRI, to differentiate between tumor and the surrounding tissues on the basis of differences in signal intensity. Hansen et al.[92] discovered that it was possible to distinguish between tissues by using different acquisition parameters.

The first images of *abnormalities* (in the brain) in living subjects were described in 1980.[93] The *thorax and abdomen* of the human body were first made visible on MR images in 1981.[9, 65] For the pelvic organs, this was achieved in 1983.[34,106-108] Thanks to the absence of motion artifacts, these last images were of excellent quality. The urinary bladder also could be displayed very well with this technique.

MRI appears to have many advantages over other imaging techniques. In particular, a comparison with the other technique that produces transverse sections of the body (CT) is important here. With MRI:
a. the image can be obtained in any plane,
b. soft tissue contrast is far better,
c. no artifacts caused by bone or air are present,
d. an image of blood vessels can be obtained without injecting contrast material and the speed of blood flow in those vessels can be studied, and
e. no use is made of ionizing radiation.

Nowadays, NMR, also called MRI, is mainly used clinically to image the contents of the skull and the extremities. More recently, however, MRI has, to an increasing extent, been used successfully to image the thorax and abdomen.

MRI appears to be a very promising imaging technique with great clinical value. In this study, an attempt is made to determine the value of MRI in patients with urinary bladder carcinoma (UBC). The goals and design of this study are described further in section 1.4.

1.2. Carcinoma of the urinary bladder

1.2.1. General aspects

Benign tumors of the urinary bladder are rare and can be subdivided into congenital (cystic) tumors, papillomas and endometriomas. The group of malignant tumors is larger.

Of the total number of carcinomas in the entire body, 4.5% are located in the urinary bladder. In the Netherlands, every year there are 2900 cases of UBC, making it the most frequent urologic malignant tumor in the country. The annual mortality in the Netherlands is high, amounting to 1000 patients. The disorder occurs more often in men than in women (male/female ratio = 7/2). Risk factors are smoking, schistosomiasis, and contact with β-naphthylamine, xenylamine (used in the dye and rubber industry), and benzidine (industry and laboratories).

To allow a comparison between therapy and diagnostics, the International Union Against Cancer (UICC) has introduced a TNM staging system for UBC.[215] Here, distinction is made between pre therapeutic, clinical TNM staging (see Table 1A) and a post operative histopathologic p.TNM staging (see Table 1B). In addition to this, a histopathologic (G) staging system has been defined (see Table 1C). Local expansion of UBC (T stages) is shown in Fig. 1-1.

The treatment and prognosis of UBC is largely determined by the depth of growth and the degree of metastasis that has occurred especially in the regional lymph nodes. The histopathological classification is also of importance here.
According to Jewett,[119] the 5-year survival rate for patients with tumors staged as T1 or T2 with a low degree of malignancy (G1-G2) is 58%, and for patients with the same tumors with a high degree of malignancy (G3), it is 48%. For patients with more deeply deeper infiltrated tumors (stages T3 and T4) the 5-year survival rate is the same for both histopathologic classification groups (16% and 15%). There is also a relationship between depth of growth, histopathologic classification and the occurrence of metastases. In patients who have a stage T1 or T2 tumor with a low degree of malignancy, Jewett[119] found no metastases, whereas in 20% of the patients with tumors of the same T stage and a high degree of malignancy metastases were found. In tumors

Table 1 A   Clinical staging with the TNM system [215].

T stages:	primary tumor
Tis	Preinvasive carcinoma (carconoma in situ)
Ta	Papillar noninvasine carcinoma.
T0	No indication of carcinoma.
T1	Palpation reveals a fairly movable tumor: however, after complete transurethral resection, this tumor should no longer be palpable, *and/or* microscopic examination should not be able to detect invasion further than the lamina propria.
T2	A mobile induration can be palpated; this has disappeared after complete transurethral resection *and/or* microscopic invasion of the superficial muscle layer can be seen.
T3	An induration or a nodular, mobile tumor mass can be palpated (by bimanual examination); this does not disappear on transurethral resection of the exophytic part of the tumor *and/or* there is microscopic invasion of the deeper muscle layer (stage T3A) or through the bladder wall (stage T3B).
T4	The tumor is fixed within or extends into the surrounding organs *and/or* there is microscopic invasion of the prostate, uterus or vagina (stage T4A) or invasion of the pelvic cavity or abdominal wall (stage T4B).
Tx	Even the minimal requirements for staging the primary tumor cannot be satisfied.

N stages:	regional or juxtaregional lymph nodes
N0	No indication of lymph node metastasis.
N1	Metastases in one ipsilateral regional lymph node.
N2	Metastases in several regional lymph nodes (contralateral or bilateral).
N3	Metastases in lymph nodes, as a result of which they become attached to the pelvic cavity.
N4	Metastases in juxtaregional lymph nodes.
Nx	Even the minimal requirements for staging of the regional or juxtaregional lymph nodes cannot be satisfied.

M stages	distant metastases
M0	No distant metastases.
M1	Distant metastases.
Mx	Even the minimal requirements for assessing whether there are distant metastases cannot be satisfied.

Table 1 B   Postoperative histopathologic (p.TNM) staging [215]

pTis	Preinvasive tumor (carcinoma in situ).
pTa	Papillar tumor; no invasion of the urothelium.
pT0	Histologic examination does not reveal any malignant tumor.
pT1	Tumor invasion limited to the lamina propria.
pT2	Tunor invasion limited to the superficial muscle layer.
pT3A	Tumor invasion limited to the deep muscle layer.
pT3B	Tumor invasion limited to the perivesical fat.
pT4A	Tumor extends into the perivesical organs and/or rectum.
pT4B	Tumor extends into the pelvic cavity or abdominal wall rectum.
pN	See Table 1A.
pM	See Table 1B.

Table 1 C   Histopathologic (G) staging [215].

G0	Papilloma: no indication of malignant tumor or atypia.
G1	High degree of differentiation.
G2	Medium degree of differentiation.
G3	Low degree of differentiation or undifferentiated tumors.
Gx	Grade cannot be assessed.

that deeply penetrate the wall of the bladder (stage T3A), the 5-years survival rate was 0% for low and 40% for high degree of malignancy. For even more deeply infiltrated tumors (as far as the perivesical fat, or stage T3B), this percentage was 36 for low and 63% for high degree of malignancy. Lymphogenous metastasis is seen earlier and more often than hematogenous metastasis.[68]

Conservative (bladder-sparing) treatment is used for superficial tumors, whereas for deeply infiltrated tumors, or once conservative treatment has failed, a radical intervention (cystectomy), and/or radiation therapy and/or chemotherapy are necessary.[68]

In the St. Radboud and the Canisius-Wilhelmina Hospitals in Nijmegen, treatment was initiated during the period of investigation mainly according to the ICE (Integral Cancer Centre, East of The Netherlands) guidelines. According to these guidelines, patients who have tumors of staged as Ta or T1 with a low degree of malignancy (G1 or G2) undergo local resection, followed by intravesical instillation of chemotherapeutics or bacille Calmette Guérin therapy[157] under meticulous cystoscopic control.

In patients who have tumors with a high degree of malignancy (G3) or in cases in which the tumor has infiltrated the muscle layer of the bladder wall (stages T2 and T3A), radiotherapy (40 Gy) is used first. If the tumor responds well to this i.e., when a second resection is performed after 40 Gy of radiation and no tumorous tissue is found, an additional doses of 26 Gy is given. The radiotherapy is then considered to have cured the patient. If the tumor does not react or incompletely reacts to 40 Gy, radical cystectomy and lymphadenectomy are performed to cure the patient.

In patients in whom the tumor has grown through the bladder wall (stage T3B), an attempt is made to achieve a cure by a combination of radiotherapy and radical surgery, but often this is no longer possible. In patients with tumor invasion of surrounding structures (stages T4A and T4B) and in patients with lymph node metastases or distant metastases, healing is no longer possible, so palliative radiotherapy or chemotherapy is used.

From the above discussion, it follows that an exact TNM and histopathologic staging system is important for prognosis and subsequent treatment of UBC.

1.2.2   Clinical staging method

In order to obtain a uniform pretherapeutic staging system in 1978, the UICC suggested a method of clinical staging for determining the T, N and M stages.[215] This method of clinical staging consists of:

For T staging:

a. clinical examination,
b. cystoscopy,
c. bimanual palpation under anesthesia before and after transurethral resection,
d. tumor resection with fractionated biopsies and
e. intravenous urography (IVU).

For N staging:

a. clinical examination,
b. radiologic studies (lymphography, IVU).

For M staging:

a. clinical examination,
b. radiologic investigation (chest radiograph; as indicated: lung planigraphy, ultrasound and/or CT of the liver, scintigraphy of the skeleton).

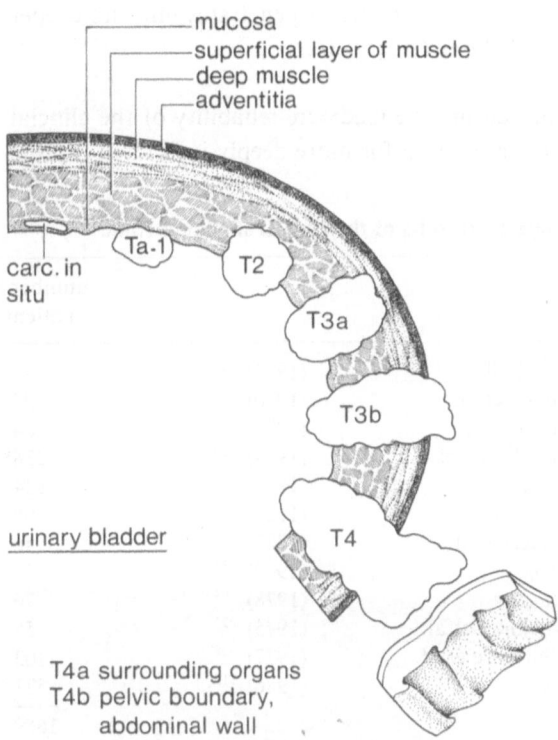

T4a surrounding organs
T4b pelvic boundary,
        abdominal wall

Fig. 1-1. T stage according to the TNM classification.[215]

In 1987, a few changes were made in the TNM staging system and the method of clinical staging.[216] As the 1978[215] system was used throughout the period of study, these changes are not pertinent here.

Table 2 summarizes the published results of the clinical staging method for UBC. The reliability (percentage correct stagings) of this method appears to be strongly dependent on the operator. Thus, it is of great importance in which way and how deep the transurethral biopsy is performed during cystoscopy and in which way and how accurately the biopsy material obtained is examined histologically. According to several authors [14, 115, 135, 164, 223, 228], the staging of superficial tumors (stages Ta-T1) is good. The accuracy of the clinical staging method for tumors staged as T2-T4 is, however, poor.[152, 202] This can probably be explained by the fact that because of the danger of perforation, the transurethral biopsy sample must not/cannot be taken deeper than the muscle layer of the bladder wall. Differentiation between stages T3A and higher is thus impossible. One exception to this is tumor invasion of the prostate (stage T4A). The differentiation between stages T2 and T3A is also difficult, because on the basis of resected tissue, the pathologist can not determine if the tumor growth is restricted to the superficial muscle layer (stage T2) or whether it penetrates into the deeper muscle layer (stage T3A).

Considering the mediocre reliability of the clincial staging method for more deeply infiltrated tumors (stages ≤ T3A), it is important to search for other, more accurate methods. These methods also should provide a more objective measure of tumor response to treatment, similar to the measures of response after for example chemotherapy or radiotherapy.

1.3 Diagnostic imaging of carcinoma of the urinary bladder

In addition to the clinical staging method, the following imaging techniques can be helpful in staging UBC:
- ultrasound (transabdominal, intravesical, and transrectal) (section 1.3.2),
- CT (section 1.3.3),
- MRI (section 1.3.5).

These radiologic methods of investigation, as well as IVU (section 1.3.1) and lymphography (section 1.3.4), which are considered to be methods of clinical staging, are discussed in the following sections.

1.3.1 Intravenous urography

Because the bladder wall itself is not visualized, it is not possible by means of IVU to determine whether a tumor has grown in or through the wall of the urinary bladder. Only the bladder lumen and protrusions in the bladder wall are visible on IVU. One can obtain information about kidney function, the renal pelvis, and the ureters via IVU. Because UBC tends to occur multifocally, it is important to rule out tumor in these areas using IVU. IVU also is useful in

Table 2   Results of the clinical staging method.

		number of patients	% correct stagings	% over-stagings	% under-stagings
Marshall	(1952) [152]	96	47	9	44
Kenny et al.	(1970) [124]	105	44	23	33
Prout et al.	(1971) [179]	104	53	13	34
Varkarakis et al.	(1974) [218]	238*	86	5	9
Richie et al.	(1975) [189]	134	34	26	40
Essed et al.	(1980) [68]	98	43-48	10-24	18
Bartels et al.	(1983) [14]	46	89	0	11
Lang	(1969) [135]	30	64	30	6
Murphy	(1978) [164]	76	51	12	37
Wasjman et al.	(1975) [223]	58	42	41	17
Whitmore et al.	(1977) [228]	103	75	6	19
Jäger et al.	(1986) [115]	571	33	—	—
		1659	33-89	0-41	6-44

* These were superficial tumors.

showing possible ureter obstruction due to tumor growth at the site of the ostium in the bladder wall. The IVU is not a reliable means of detecting urinary bladder tumors. Using this technique, Schmidt and Weinstein[202] only found a filling defect in 40% of their patients with urinary bladder tumor. Hillman et al.[103] were somewhat more successful with IVU recognizing tumors in a maximum of only 60% of their patients with urinary bladder tumor.

In summary: IVU is valuable in pretherapeutic examination of patients with UBC. IVU is not, however, suitable for detection and staging of the UBC.

1.3.2   Ultrasound

With the introduction of ultrasound, a new method of investigation was introduced in the field of medical imaging. We can distinguish three methods for diagnosing urinary bladder tumors:
1. transabdominal (suprapubic) ultrasound,
2. transrectal ultrasound, and
3. intravesicular ultrasound.

A literature review of the staging accuracy of ultrasound is presented in Table 3. The accuracy of both transabdominal and intravesicular ultrasound shows a certain amount of variability. The reason for this is probably the large degree of observer dependence.

A disadvantage of *all* ultrasound techniques when investigating the urinary bladder is that they cannot distinguish malignant urinary bladder tumors from chronic cystitis, local hypertrophy of the bladder wall, or blood clots.[1, 56, 101] Furthermore, on the basis of sonographic criteria, it is not possible to distinguish between superficial and deep invasion of the bladder wall.[56, 114, 191] It is precisely this distinction that some clinics consider important for the choice of therapy. In patients with tumors staged as T1 and in some with tumors staged as T2, local resection is sufficient, whereas in patients with tumors staged as T3A, cystectomy is usually performed.

The value of ultrasound is very limited in the determination of lymph node metastases. To show 'distant' metastases (liver metastases), transabdominal ultrasound is of value.[19, 36, 86, 143, 213]

Transabdominal ultrasound is indeed not an invasive investigation, but it is not always possible to produce a good image of the urinary bladder. Denkhaus et al.[56] did not manage to obtain a good sonographic image of the urinary bladder in 11 (10%) of 112 patients. They did not, therefore, include those patients is their final results. Reasons why ultrasound was not successful in these patients were apparently scars on the stomach wall as a result of previous operations, radiotherapy, and poor filling of the bladder because of dysuria or adipositas. The accuracy of transabdominal ultrasound in the staging UBC is mediocre (61-84%, see Table 3).

It appears from Table 3 that *transrectal ultrasound* is rarely used in staging UBC. With transrectal ultrasound, it is possible to produce good images of the bladder neck and the trigonum vesicae. However, tumors in the bladder dome and the anterior wall of the bladder are poorly visualized. The accuracy of transrectal ultrasound is comparable to that of transabdominal ultrasound.

Intravesical ultrasound gains the highest score with regard to reliability: 62-92% (see Table 3). This is particularly the case for superficial tumors[5, 32, 101, 172]. Previously reported limitations of ultrasound such as the inability to differentiate between malignant tumors, inflammation, local hypertrophy of the wall, and a blood clot, or between tumor stages T2 and T3A,[101, 167, 191, 203] also apply here. Furthermore, staging by this technique is unreliable for large tumors ($\leq$ 3 cm) because of the 'shadow' cast by the tumor mass. This often results in overstaging.[115] Moreover, intravesicular ultrasound is an invasive technique that has to be performed with the patient under general anesthesia. Because cystoscopic examination *with* intravesicular ultrasound takes longer and special equipment has to be introduced into the bladder, the chance of infection is greater than with cystoscopy alone.[85]

In summary: intravesicular ultrasound is an asset for staging local growth of UBC (T stages). Transabdominal and transrectal ultrasound have their limitations. In cases of large tumors ($\leq$ 3 cm)and tumors that have infiltrated the wall deeply, even intravesicular ultrasound is only moderately reliable. Differentiation between malignant infiltration, inflammation, hypertrophy of the wall and blood clots cannot be achieved with ultrasound. The value of ultrasound in staging lymph node metastases of UBC (N stages) is limited.

1.3.3   Computed tomography

For the determination of T, N and M stages, CT is also used nowadays. In the following section, the three categories of UBC will be dealt with individually.

T staging:

At the end of the 1970s, CT was first used as an additional method for pre operative staging of UBC.[205,206] Since then, many publications have appeared concerning the reliability of this technique (Table 4). The percentage of correct stagings of local growth of UBC (T stages) by CT is 40-92%. These numbers could not be improved by the use of other agents, such as filling the bladder with positive and/or negative contrast agents.[4, 91, 102, 161, 167, 197] Table 4 conveys the reliability of CT only for differentiating between tumor stages Ta-T3A, T3B, T4A, and T4B. Because CT cannot differentiate between stages Ta, T1, T2 and T3A (all authors in Table 4 but Ahlberg et al.[4]), these stages have been combined into one (Ta-T3A). The numbers in this table, therefore, only show the accuracy of CT in determining the degree of *extravesicular* tumor growth. The only authors who attempt to differentiate tumors staged as T_2 from those staged as T3A are Ahlberg et al.[4] The series described by them is, however, too small to allow conclusions to be drawn.

Another limitation of CT is the inability to distinguish tumor tissue from other causes of local thickening of the bladder wall, as seen in cases of bladder wall hypertrophy, local inflammation and fibrosis. Local inflammation of the bladder wall results from earlier tumor resection or radiotherapy. Staging of tumors by using CT after the patient has undergone radiotherapy or transurethral tumor resection is thus less reliable. It is mainly because of this that overstaging occurs more often with CT than does understaging (see Table 4).

Another disadvantage of CT is the limitation that suitable images can be obtained only in the transverse plane. This makes it particularly difficult to assess the depth of tumor invasion in the dome or base of the bladder.[123, 167, 197] Also, because of the 'partial volume' effect, it can be difficult to establish possible invasion of nearby organs (e.g., vesiculae seminales).[205] The use of sagittal and coronal reconstruction methods does not help.[91]

N staging:

Many publications exist concerning the reliability of CT in showing lymph node metastases (see Table 5). The values quoted vary from 50% to 97%. It is apparent from these numbers that CT is certainly valuable in N staging. However, this technique also has its limitations:
-   small nodes with microscopic metastases are not recognized as being abnormal,
-   considering the fact that it is only by the size of the lymph nodes on the CT scan that lymph node metastases are assessed, it is not possible to distinguish between benign hypertrophy of the lymph node and lymph node enlargement caused by metastases,
-   differentiation between bowel loops and lymph nodes is sometimes difficult with CT, and
-   problems often occur with the differentiation between blood vessels and lymph nodes. Administration of intravenous contrast material is then necessary.

M staging:

Lung metastases can easily be detected with CT: however, lung tomography is cheaper and just as effective.[18, 122, 176] Liver metastases can be traced well with CT, but ultrasound is cheaper and just as reliable.[19, 25, 36, 86, 142] Bone and bone marrow metastases can be shown radiologically only once bone destruction has appeared. Bone scintigraphy is a more sensitive method and is thus used more often.[25, 51]

In summary: CT is a valuable addition to the clinical staging method because it allows determination extravesicular tumor growth and the presence of pathologically enlarged lymph nodes.

1.3.4 Lymphography

Bipedal lymphography is a method frequently used to visualize primary or secondary malignant tumors of the pelvic lymph nodes. There is no doubt about the accuracy of the staging of malignant lymphoma: it is high (90% correct stagings).[121, 134, 148, 183] With regard to its reliability for determining metastases in malignant tumors in the pelvis, opinions are divided. In the literature, the percentage of correct stagings varies from 79% to 94% (see Table 6). This is probably because both the way the investigation is

Table 3   Results of staging with ultrasound (T-stages).

		number of patients	% correct stagings		
			transabdominal sonography	transrectal sonography	intravesical sonography
Denkhaus et al.	(1985) [56]	65	84	—	—
Rozsahegyi et al.	(1985) [191]	100	61	69	92
Schüller et al.	(1982) [203]	28	—	—	92
Itzack et al.	(1981) [114]	27	67	—	—
Abu-Yousef et al.	(1984) [1]	14	79	—	—
Resnick et al.	(1986) [187]	62	—	—	84
Jäger et al.	(1986) [115]	571	—	—	70
Alzin et al.	(1983) [5]	190	—	—	88
Braeckman et al.	(1983) [32]	72	—	—	83
Greiner et al.	(1983) [85]	25	—	—	64
Janetschek et al.	(1983) [116]	41	—	—	86
Pfitzermaier et al.	(1982) [174]	31	—	—	65
Paoletti et al.	(1982) [172]	18	—	—	89
Schmidtbauer et al.	(1983) [201]	44	—	—	86
Nicolas et al.	(1988) [167]	32	—	—	62
Hendriks et al.	(1989) [101]	15	—	—	73
		1335	61-84	69	62-92

Table 4   Results of staging with CT (T stages).

		number of patients	% correct stagings	% over-stagings	% under-stagings
Siedelmann et al.	(1977) [205]	21	81	19	0
Siedelmann et al.	(1978) [206]	21	86	14	0
Yu et al.	(1979) [234]	17	88	6	6
Kellet et al.	(1980) [123]	15	80	13	7
Frödin et al.	(1981) [80]	12	80	17	0
Koss et al.	(1981) [130]	25	64	20	16
Morgan et al.	(1981) [161]	25	92	—	—
Ahlberg et al.	(1982) [4]	9	89	11	0
Vock et al.	(1982) [220]	35	81	18	1
Weinermann et al.	(1982) [225]	33	64	21	15
Bartels et al.	(1983) [14]	50	76	22	2
Greiner et al.	(1983) [85]	28	78	18	4
Sager et al.	(1983) [197]	32	78	22	0
Engelmann et al.	(1984) [67]	74	64	26	10
Salo et al.	(1985) [198]	103	66	25	9
Nicolas et al.	(1988) [167]	161	82	12	6
Amendola et al.	(1986) [6]	10	40	50	10
Rholl et al.	(1987) [188]	19	85	5	15
Bryan et al.	(1987) [35]	13	69	8	23
Fisher et al.	(1985) [76]	12	64	12	24
Barentsz et al.	(1987) [13]	24	71	8	21
Buy et al.	(1988) [43]	30	60	3	37
		769	40-92	3-50	0-37

performed and its interpretation are highly investigator dependent.

Since the introduction of CT, various studies have been published about the reliability of both these methods[72, 117, 130, 138] (see also section 1.3.3). Apparently CT is of greater value in cases of massive lymph node metastases, whereas lymphography is better for tracing small localized foci in normal-sized nodes.[59, 130, 138, 177, 212]

In summary: lymphography is an accurate method of investigation for the determination of lymph node metastases. An advantage over CT is that this technique also can detect small metastases in normal-sized nodes.

1.3.5 Magnetic Resonance Imaging

In 1983, images obtained by using MRI were found to be equal in quality to CT images. This was particularly true for the brain, the spinal cord, and the extremities. MRI of the thorax and abdomen was more problematic. Because of the long acquisition time, motion artifacts were present because of breathing, heartbeat, intestinal peristalsis, and the patient's random movements. Nevertheless, MRI did provide useful information about abdominal organs. This was particularly valid for retroperitoneal structures.[108, 159]

Because motion artifacts in the pelvis are minimal, MR images of the pelvis proved to be of better quality than those of the thorax and the upper abdomen.[34, 42, 95, 106, 107, 112] The first publications on MRI in UBC appeared in 1983.[34, 106, 107] Local growth of the carcinoma could be established very reliably by using MRI. The determination of lymph node metastases was, conversely, less accurate. Since that time, more publications have appeared, which emphasize the significant improvements in staging of UBC.

Table 7 summarizes published data on the accuracy of MRI compared with that of CT in the T and N staging of UBC. The accuracy of MRI for *T staging* varies from 73% to 96%. These values are 10-33% higher than those obtained with CT. With MRI it is also possible to distinguish between stages T_2 and T3A, something that is not possible with either ultrasound or CT.[11, 13, 43, 76, 188]

In *N staging* MRI and CT are equal: the percentage of correct stagings for CT is 83-97% versus 73-98% for MRI.

Little is known about the value of MRI for *M staging*. For determination of lung metastases, lung planigraphy is still the indicated imaging technique.[18, 122, 176] Ultrasound (if necessary supplemented by CT) is the preferred method for showing liver metastases.[19, 25, 36, 86, 143, 213] Bone scintigraphy is currently the method of choice for detecting bone (marrow) metastases.[51] The sensitivity of MRI in showing bone marrow metastases appears, however, to be greater than that of scintigraphy.[49]

In summary: on the basis of data currently available in the literature, MRI seems to be the most accurate imaging technique for staging local growth (T stages) of UBC. Lymph node metastases (N stages) also can be well established with MRI. Finally, MRI also may have advantages for the detection of bone marrow metastases (M stages).

1.4. Aims and design of this study

Both the number of MRI studies carried out on UBC and the number of patients investigated by MRI is fairly limited (see Table 7). A description of the factors that lead to optimal visualization of UBC with MRI and of the normal MR image of the urinary bladder and surrounding organs does not appear in the literature.

This study was designed precisely because the staging of UBC with MRI seems to be so promising. The aim is to answer the following questions:

1. What is the *optimal MR technique* (parameters) for imaging the urinary bladder?
2. What does the *normal anatomy* of the urinary bladder look like on MRI?
3. How is *UBC* displayed on MRI?
4. What is the *value of MRI* in cases of UBC?
5. Can MRI replace other, *existing staging techniques*?

With this in mind, **Chapter 2** deals with the general principles of MRI. After a short introduction, the text discusses the pulse sequences to be used and factors that can influence the imaging. Finally, this chapter also considers advantages and disadvantages, safety aspects and contraindications for MRI.

Table 5   Results of staging with CT (N stages).

		number of patients	% correct stagings
Lee et al.	(1978) [138]	26	73
Walsh et al.	(1980) [222]	8	50
Koss et al.	(1981) [130]	25	92
Bartels et al.	(1983) [14]	19	95
Weinerman et al.	(1982) [225]	13	92
Hodson et al.	(1979) [105]	36	81
Vock et al.	(1982) [220]	44	89
Morgan et al.	(1981) [161]	34	79
Nicolas et al.	(1988) [167]	40	85
Amendola et al.	(1986) [6]	10	90
Rholl et al.	(1987) [188]	19	95
Bryan et al.	(1987) [35]	9	89
Barentsz et al.	(1987) [13]	112	83
Buy et al.	(1988) [43]	30	97
		325	50-97

Table 6   Results of staging with lymfography.

		number of patients	% correct stagings
Wasjman et al.	(1975) [223]	18	94
Johnson et al.	(1979) [120]	49	90
Strijk et al.	(1983) [212]	19	89
Hodson et al.	(1979) [105]	36	81
Vock et al.	(1982) [220]	44	89
Morgan et al.	(1981) [161]	34	79
Nicolas et al.	(1988) [167]	40	85
Barentsz et al.	(1987) [13]	10	90
		250	79-94

Table 7   Results of staging with CT and MRI (T and N stages).

		CT			MRI		
		number of patients	% correct T stagings	% correct N stagings	number of patients	% correct T stagings	% correct N stagings
Koebel et al.	(1988) [126]	—	—	—	10	90	—
Amendola et al.	(1986) [6]	10	40	90	11	73	91
Küper et al.	(1986) [131]	15	—	—	12	75	—
Fisher et al.	(1985) [76]	12	64	—	14	85	—
Rholl et al.	(1987) [188]	19	85	95	23	96	96
Bryan et al.	(1987) [35]	9	67	89	10	80	90
Beyer et al.	(1985) [20]	—	—	—	26	80	73
Nicolas et al.	(1988) [167]	161	82	—	13	92	—
Barentsz et al.	(1987) [13]	24	71	83	24	92	83
Barentsz et al.	(1988) [11]	24	—	—	24	92	88
Buy et al.	(1988) [43]	30	60	97	40	83	98
			40-85	83-97		73-96	73-98

In **Chapter 3** the technical factors involved in MRI examination are described, concentrating on patients with UBC. Patient related factors and their influence on image quality also are described. Which pulse sequences are best for imaging UBC are determined. Improvement in image quality by using a surface coil is evaluated. At the end of Chapter 3, results obtained with a weaker magnetic field (0.5 T) are compared with those from a stronger magnetic field (1.5 T).

With a view to facilitating the interpretation of abnormal images, **Chapter 4** first presents a correlation of the normal MR image of the pelvis with anatomic data. Of essence here is a comparison between the MR images and an anatomic preparation of the pelvis and of cystectomy preparations.

Chapter 5 deals with the value of MRI in the staging of patients with UBC. Results of the MRI study are compared with those from a CT study. The main reference values are the histopathologic findings after cystectomy. The findings of the clinical staging method (including follow-up for an average of 18 months) also are compared with the results of MRI and CT.

In **Chapter 6**, conclusions are drawn and a brief discussion is presented of new developments in MR that are important in the MR imaging of UBC.

II

GENERAL PRINCIPLES OF MRI

2.1 Introduction

Nuclear magnetic resonance (NMR) is a form of spectroscopy that can be used to gain information about the composition of certain substances. This involves measuring the characteristic spectrum of various substances or tissues. This spectrum can be used to determine the presence and relative concentration of that particular substance and to establish the molecular structure.

This has led to the current use in medicine of *MRS (magnetic resonance spectroscopy)* to study ischemia of muscle[168, 169] and brain tissue. Experiments also have been performed that have shown differences in energy metabolism between tumor tissue in the breast and normal breast tissue.[54]

In addition to MRS, NMR is used to produce an image of various structures and parts of the body. Imaging by means of NMR is called *magnetic resonance imaging (MRI)*. Nowadays, the medical world mainly uses MRI; while in vivo application of MRS is still in its infancy.

In an effort to understand how this image is created, the basic concepts about MRI will be dealt with in the following sections. MRS is beyond the scope of this book. During the last few years, many publications have appeared that describe the general principles of MRI.[81, 99, 171, 207, 217] Because of their complexity, the basic principles of MRI often seem confusing even to those who are at home in the field of physics. It is essential that the general radiodiagnostician understand what makes 'black structures black and white structures white' on MR images. MRI handbooks[64, 81, 97-99, 171, 207, 217] should be consulted for more detailed information.

Although at first glance, the final result of MRI, a *spin image*, looks like a conventional radiologic image, MRI is based on completely different principles from all other imaging techniques. Other radiologic techniques detect bending of X-rays and produce an image by means of projection and reflection. On the contrary, in MRI the image is formed by the signal emitted by the *nuclear spin* itself. The wavelength of the MR 'radiation' spans several meters and does not bear any relation to the final resolution of the image. The radiofrequency 'radiation' used, is low in energy, and in contrast to other imaging techniques where ionizing radiation is used, cannot result in radiation damage (see also section 2.8).

2.2 Basic physics of MRI

2.2.1 Nuclear spins, resonant frequency

Atomic nuclei show a rotational movement *(nuclear spin)*. In atomic nuclei that have an uneven number of protons and/or neutrons, this results in a magnetic moment; this means they can be regarded as small bar magnets (magnetic dipoles). Atoms with an even number of protons and/or neutrons do not possess this magnetic property, and are therefore not suitable for MRI. In living organisms, there are only a limited number of naturally occurring elements whose atomic nuclei contain an uneven number of protons and/or neutrons and thus make NMR possible. These are: 1H (1 proton, no neutrons) 13C (6 protons, 7 neutrons) 23Na (11 protons, 12 neutrons) 31P (15 protons and 16 neutrons).

The human body consists largely of water and fat, substances that contain a high proportion of hydrogen nuclei (protons). Hence, in performing MRI of the human body, use is made of protons.

In the absence of an externally applied magnetic field, the direction of the magnetic dipoles is random. This results in a net magnetism of zero. Conversely, in a strong magnetic field, the magnetic dipoles adopt a fixed orientation: slightly more than half the protons are aligned with and the rest are aligned opposite the external field. As a result of the Brownian movements and the magnetic interaction between nearby molecules, the magnetic dipoles flip constantly back and forth between the parallel and antiparallel state. This results in a very small magnetization in the direction of the external magnetic field.

As the magnetic dipoles align themselves, the nuclei show rotational movement around the directional axis of the main field. This movement is called *precession*. It appears that the speed of precession, also called *precession or resonant frequency*, is directly proportional to the strength of the magnetic field and depends on a physical constant that is specific for every isotope, the *gyromagnetic ratio*.

The principle of MRI lies in disturbing the distribution of parallel and antiparallel orientations by applying so much energy to the magnetic dipoles that they change orientation. The amount of energy necessary for transition from the one state to the other depends on resonant frequency. In practice, one supplies energy by 'radiating' a short electromagnetic radio-frequency (RF) pulse perpendicular to the external magnetic field. Here, the frequency of the RF pulse must be equal to the precession frequency, so that the spins can resonate. As a result of the RF pulse, magnetization is created perpendicular to the direction of the magnetic field. For a short time after this pulse, the magnetic dipoles relax and adopt their original state. This produces a detectable MR signal that contains valuable information about the nuclear-spins and their environment. This MR signal is ultimately used to create the image.

The frequencies of the RF pulse and the MR signal lie in the range of FM radio waves. For proton spin imaging, this varies for currently used magnets (0.5-2.0 T) between 10 and 85 MHz.

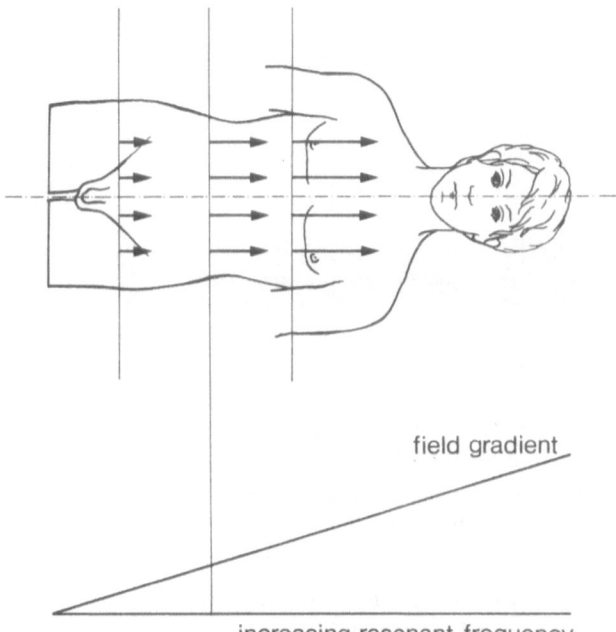

field gradient

increasing resonant frequency

Fig. 2-1. There is a gradient along the longitudinal axis of the patient, along which the resonant frequency per plane varies perpendicularly.

2.2.2 Spin imaging: proton density, T_1 and T_2 relaxation times

When generating an MR image for medical purposes, use is made of the signal emitted by protons. Differences in proton density and in mutual interactions between the protons give rise to contrasts that ensure that the tissue structures in the body can be differentiated.

To generate an MR image, it is essential to determine the site where a particular proton density can be found. Such information can be obtained by virtue of the fact that the resonance frequency depends on the strength of the magnetic field.

When an extra coil elicits a second, extra magnetic field, which is not homogeneous but which differs in strength from place to place, every nuclear spin at a different site will experience a different magnetic field strength. This means that at each site the resonant frequency will also be slightly different. Fig. 2-1 shows this gradient, that is, a decrease of the magnetic field from one end of the patient to the other. Within one slice of the body, all nuclear spins will have the same resonant frequency, because they are all subjected to the same magnetic field strength. Thus, as a result of a correct RF (90°) pulse, all spins in a 'selected' slice will be excited. In order to be able to separate individual points in this slice (X, Y), it is essential to use two other field gradients. In the Y

direction, as soon as the excitation pulse is over and all spins are in resonance, a third magnetic field, the *preparation gradient*, is introduced for a short time. This results in the positions of the separate points in the Y direction becoming linearly related to the phase of the precession of the magnetization vector.

After this, a fourth magnetic field, the *readout* gradient, is introduced in the X direction of the slice. This will cause the resonating spins whose balance has been disturbed to rotate with different precession frequencies. For some this means that the precession frequency remains the same. For others it becomes a little slower or faster. The result is that the spectrum received will contain a whole series of frequencies. Every frequency component represents a column in the slice. The intensity of the frequency component is proportional to the number of hydrogen spins present in the column. In other words: the proton density has now been established along a number of lines.

If the slice is now excited a few times in succession and then a stronger Y gradient used, it is possible to reconstruct an image of the cross section from all the line measurements. With the help of a mathematical technique, the *two dimensional Fourier transformation*,[69] a computer can calculate a cross sectional image in a matter of seconds.

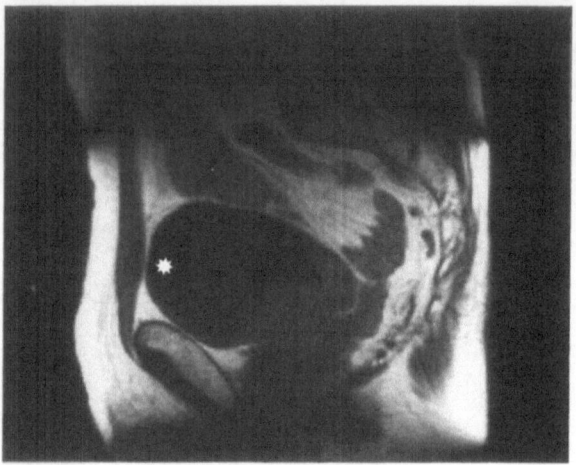 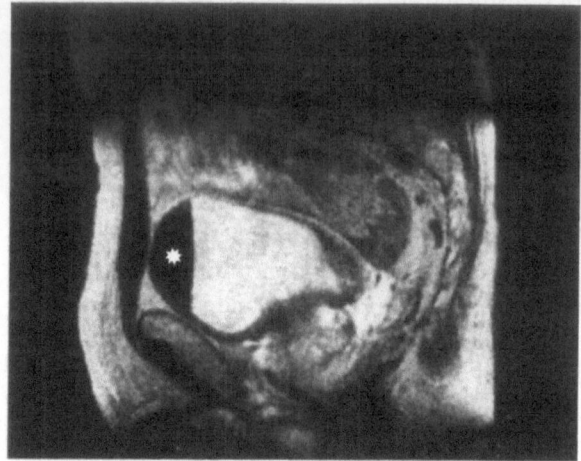

Fig. 2-2. On sagittal MR images (a) (0.5 T; SE/750/30/2) and (b) (0,5 T; SE/2000/150/2), the air ventral in the bladder (*), just as the cortex of the pubic bone, gives no signal.

After the transformation, every point on the image corresponds to a certain frequency. The size of the frequency component decides the intensity. By translating the intensities into certain gray values or colours, the final MR image emerges. High signal intensities appear white.

Every pixel (picture element) in this image corresponds to the MR signal of one volume element (voxel), bounded on three sides, of the part of the body under investigation. Using the above described gradient system in the X, Y, and Z directions, one can produce an image of a thin slice (only a few millimeters thick) of a certain part of the body in any direction one wants.

The tissue contrast, the difference in gray values between the various points of an MR image, is a reflection of the differences in MR signal strength. In the first instance, the signal intensity depends on the concentration of nuclear spins *(proton density)* in the volume element concerned. The differences in proton density of the various tissue types in the human body are very small. If based solely on these differences in concentration, the MR image would contain little relevant information. Only tissues with very few protons will demonstrate such a low signal that they can easily be distinguished. This is the case with bone cortex, air, tendons and calcifications (Fig. 2-2). The contrast in the MR image is further determined by a pair of typical tissue properties: the *spin relaxation times, T_1 and T_2*. Once the nuclear spins have lost their balance orientation because of

an RF pulse (Fig. 2-3b), it takes a while before all spins have returned to their original situation. We call this process *relaxation*; the duration of the process is the *relaxation time*. This relaxation is characterized by two parameters (Fig. 2-3c and 2-3d).

If one looks at the recovery of the magnetization of the spins in the direction of the external field (Fig. 2-3c), then one is considering the first parameter. The exponential recovery of the magnetization in this longitudinal direction is characterized by the T_1 *or longitudinal relaxation time*. Because this recovery is the result of interactions between the individual spins and the nearby molecules in the lattice, this is also called the *spin lattice relaxation time*. T_1 is defined as the time that is necessary for the recovery of almost two thirds (63%) of the longitudinal magnetization. T_1 is characteristic of the type of tissue. Molecules with a large freedom of movement, such as in water or in urine, contain nuclear spins with a long T_1. Nuclear spins with a limited freedom of movement, such as the 'bound' protons in fat, are characterized by a much shorter T_1. T_1 depends on field strength: as the strength of the field increases, T_1 becomes longer.[28]

After the RF pulse, magnetization arises in the plane of this pulse. As the latter is applied at right angles to the external field, one can use the term 'transverse magnetization'. When the RF pulse is terminated, this transverse magnetization will decline rapidly. A small part of this decrease is caused by the relaxation of the proton spins in the direction of the external magnetic field (the T_1 effect). By far the greatest part of this decrease is caused by the slight difference in resonant frequency between the various spins resulting from spin-spin interactions and inhomogeneity of the external magnetic field. This is also called loss of phase coherence (Fig. 2-3d).

The degree of decrease in this magnetization in the transverse plane is characterized by the second parameter: T_2, *transverse or spin-spin relaxation time*. T_2 is the time necessary for the transverse magnetization to decrease to 37% of the level immediately after excitation. T_2 also is characteristic of the tissue type. Otherwise, T_2 is independent of the field strength used.[28,81]

The final signal measured from a certain tissue contains a part determined by T_1 and by T_2. Considering the inevitable limit to the recording time, there is usually no time between excitations to await complete recovery of the longitudinal magnetization. Therefore, tissues with a short T_1 have a larger longitudinal magnetization when the measurement is repeated (tm), than do tissues with a long T_1. Because more longitudinal relaxation leads to more signal, tissues with a short T_1 will appear 'whiter' (Fig. 2-4).

Immediately after the RF pulse, the longitudinal magnetization increases from zero to a certain maximum. Conversely, the transverse magnetization 'starts' at a maximum and then decreases. Tissues with a short T_2 lose phase coherence more rapidly and hence transverse magnetization decreases more quickly. At a certain point in time (tm), the signal from tissues with a short T_2 (e.g. fat) will, therefore, be smaller than that from tissues with a long T_2 (e.g. urine). Tissues with a short T_2 will therefore produce a darker image than tissues with a long T_2 (Fig. 2-5). The T_1 and T_2 effects can work against each other: in a tissue with short T_1 and T_2, the high signal resulting from the short T_1 is weakened by the low signal resulting from the short T_2.

The T_1 determines the *recovery process* of longitudinal magnetization, T_2 determines the process of *decrease* of transverse magnetization. The T_1 and T_2 values for various tissues allow detailed, contrast rich MR images, presenting a very accurate display of structures inside the body, to be produced within acceptable measurement times. Table 8 surveys the relationship between proton density, the T_1 and T_2 values, and the gray values in images of pelvic tissues.

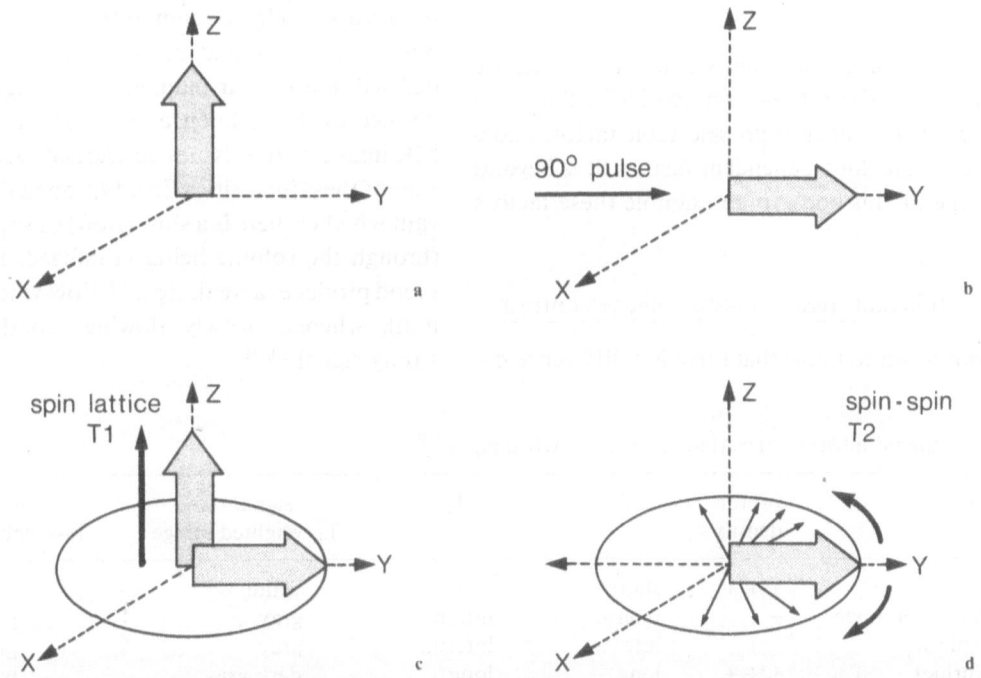

Fig. 2-3. (a) Initial balanced situation. **(b)** The magnetization is turned through 90° by a radiofrequency pulse; **(c)** and **(d)** illustrate the T1 and T2 components, respectively of the relaxation process. T1 is the speed with which the magnetization returns to the direction of the Z-axis (thick black arrow). T2 is determined by the speed with which the electron spins lose their phase coherence as a result of electromagnetic interaction with each other. Consequently, they start to turn with different speeds in the X-Y plane and the resulting magnetization decreases in the direction of the Y-axis.

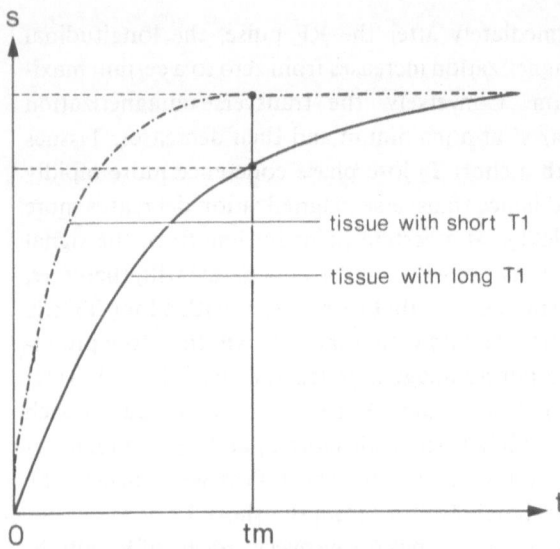

Fig. 2-4. At point in time tm, the tissue with a short T1 has a stronger signal (S) than the tissue with a longer T1.

Fig. 2-5. At point in time tm, the tissue with a long T2 has a stronger signal (S) than the tissue with a shorter T2.

2.3   Image contrast

The quality of an MR image is determined by tissue contrasts, structure definition, and the degree of noise. In the MR image, the contrast is due to a difference in signal intensity between tissues. The definition of the image is determined by the voxel size. Noise has a negative effect on the general quality of the image.

In order to measure the quality of an MR image, use is made of the *signal-to-noise ratio (SNR)*. This ratio depends on a number of pre selectable factors and a number of machine-dependent factors. It is beyond the scope of this book to go examine these factors here.

2.3.1.   'Inherent' tissue contrast, image contrast

It is important to know that there is a difference be-tween 'inherent' tissue contrast and the ultimate contrast seen on the MR image (image contrast). *Inherent tissue contrast* is determined by factors characteristic for that tissue: proton density and T_1 and T_2 values. Inherent T_1 contrast between two tissues is defined as the difference in T_1 values of the two tissues divided by the sum of these two values. Inherent T_2 contrast and proton density contrast are defined in a similar manner. The *image contrast* is defined as the difference in signal intensity on the MR image of the tissues concerned, divided by the sum of these intensities. In addition to this, it is relevant whether there is a shift (flow) of spins within or through the volume being visualized. Fast-flowing blood produces a weak signal ('flow-void' phenomenon), whereas, slowly flowing blood displays a strong signal.[30, 31]

Table 8   Signal intensity of various tissues on MR images [140].

Tissued	proton density	T_1	T_2	signal on T_1-weighted image	signal on T_2-weighted image
fat	+ + +	short	interm.	white	gray
muscle, lymph node	+ +	interm.	interm.	gray	gray
liver, spleen	+ +	interm.	interm.	gray	gray
fluid (urine)	+ + +	long	long	dark gray	white
haematoma	+ + +	short	long	white	white
bone, tendon, air	—	—	—	black	black
blood vessel	+ + +*)	—	—	black	black

*) = flowing protons.

2.3.2. Ajustable factors, pulse sequences

The setting of the adjustable factors by the MR user determines how inherent tissue contrasts can be converted into contrasts on the image. Contrast between the various tissues on an MR image can be influenced by the following adjustable factors:

a. type of pulse sequence,
b. inter pulse times: repetition time (TR), echo time (TE) and inversion time (TI),
c. angle of rotation (flip angle) (see section 6.2.3.),
d. thickness of the slice imaged,
e. field of view, and finally
f. the scale of the matrix.

Changes in slice thickness and field of view result in a change in the volume visualized. Volume changes give rise to changes in the number of protons which visualized and thus also to changes in the signal intensity. The effects of flip angle change(s) are discussed in section 6.2.3.

In the next section, an indication will be given of how the choice of the type of pulse sequence and of the sequence times influences the contrast in the MR image. The contrast in the final MR image is mainly determined by the way in which the RF energy is applied and how the signals received from the patient are interpreted. It is not only the emitted RF pulse and the signals received from the patient that are important here, but also the gradients used, necessary for the choice of slices to be imaged. Both the selected gradient and the scale of the matrix are important for image resolution. All these factors are described within the *pulse sequence*.

2.3.2.1 *Spin-echo pulse sequence*

The pulse sequence used most frequently in medical MR imaging is the *spin-echo (SE)* sequence. This sequence is reproduced schematically in Figure 2-6. In the SE sequence, an RF pulse is emitted, which causes a 90° rotation of the spin magnetization (90° pulse). A few to tens of milliseconds later (echo time: TE/2), a 180° pulse is applied. This 180° pulse causes a reversal of the dephasing of the spins in the transverse plane. An equal time period (TE/2) after the 180 pulse, a signal is reflected as a result of the rephasing. Another name sometimes applied to this signal is the *spin echo*. This signal reaches its maximum at time TE after the 90° pulse.

The 180° pulse is necessary to eliminate the dephasing effects, which are caused by inhomogeneity of the main magnetic field and the gradient fields. Thanks to this pulse, only the dephasing resulting from the spin-spin interactions is measured. Two important parameters characterize the SE sequence: the *repetition time (TR)* and the *echo time (TE)*. TR is the time interval between the 90° pulses. The TR determines to a large extent the duration of the sequences and thus the duration of the investigation. TE is twice the time that passes between the middle of the 90° pulse and the 180° pulse. For a certain voxel, the signal intensity of a certain tissue (Sse) in the MR image is given by the following formula:

$$S_{SE} = N[H].e^{-TE/T2}.(1-e^{-TR/T1}).\ [171]$$

Although this formula appears rather complicated, clearly it consists of three parts:

- the first part: *N[H]*, represents the *proton density*,
- the second part is the *T_2 factor: $e^{-TE/T2}$*,
- the third part is the *T_1 factor: $1-e^{-TR/T1}$*.

It is clear from the above that in the formula, TE appears together with T_2 and TR with T_1. This indicates that the T_2 effect on an SE image can be influ-

spin echo

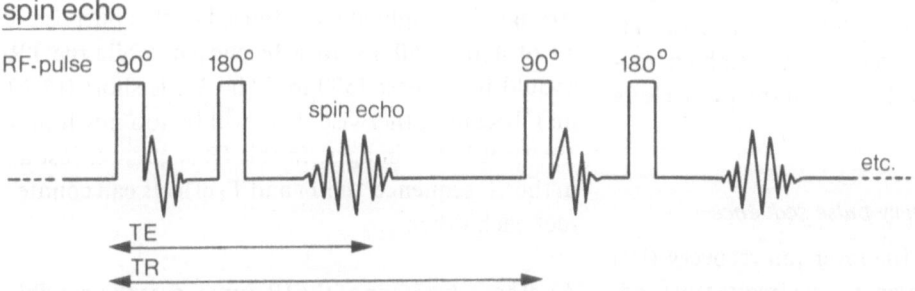

Fig. 2-6. Schematic representation of the spin echo (SE) sequence.

inversion recovery

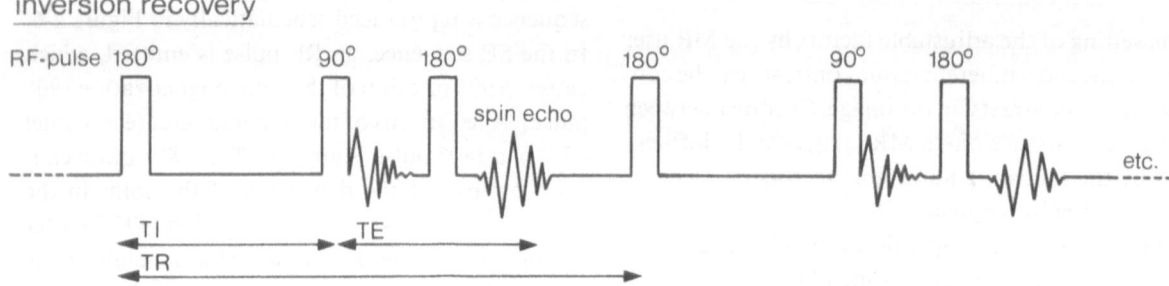

Fig. 2-7. Schematic representation of the inversion recovery (IR) sequence.

enced with the help of TE, and the T_1 effect, with the help of TR. Conversely, the effect of proton density is independent of TR and TE and is, therefore, always present at the same strength in an SE image. By varying TR and TE, it is possible to obtain an image in which the T_1 effect dominates the T_2 effect or the proton density. An image in which the T_1 effect dominates is called *T_1 dominant or T_1 weighted*. In a similar way, an image in which the T_2 effect dominates is called *T_2 dominant or T_2 weighted*. If the proton density is predominant, the image is referred to as *proton weighted*.

In the SE sequences, the T_1 and T_2 effects can counteract each other (see also section 2.2.2): a tissue with short T_1 and short T_2 has a high signal intensity as a result of the T_1 effect and a low signal intensity as a result of the T_2 effect; a tissue with a long T_1 and a long T_2 has a low signal intensity due to the T_1 and a high signal intensity due to the T_2 effect.

In general, higher spatial resolution is achieved in T_1 weighted images by a good signal-to-noise ratio. This is why these sequences are used for optimal imaging of the anatomy. The T_2 weighted images are used to improve differentiation between various tissue types. It is generally the case that with a short TR ($<$1000 ms) and a short TE ($<$30 ms), the SE image is T_1 weighted. A proton weighted image arises if the TR is long (the T_1 effect decreases) and the TE is short (the T_2 effect decreases). A T_2 weighted image is obtained with a long TR ($>$2000 ms) and a long TE ($>$60 ms).

2.3.2.2 *Inversion recovery pulse sequence*

After the SE sequence, the inversion recovery (IR) sequence is the pulse sequence most frequently used. This sequence is shown in Fig. 2-7. Here, the net spin

magnetization is first turned through 180°. Some time later *(TI = inversion time)*, the magnetization is turned through 90°, so that it can be measured.

Shortly hereafter, analogous to the SE sequence, a 180° rephasing pulse is given, after which an 'echo' can be recorded. Here too the TE is the time that passes between the 90° pulse and the maximum of the 'echo'. The TR time is the time between the initial 180° pulses of each sequence.

In these sequences, there are three parameters that can be set: TR, TE, and TI. The formula that describes the signal amplitude for the IR sequence is

$$S_{IR} = N[H].e^{-TE/T2}.(1-2e^{-TI/T1}+e^{-TR/T1}).\ ^{171}$$

Just as in the SE sequence, there is a proton-density-, a T1-, and a T2-dependent factor in the IR sequence. In IR images, the T_1 factor is, however, not only dependent on TR, but also on TI. Just as in the SE sequence, the T_2 factor is *only* dependent on the TE.

An advantage of the IR sequence is the fact that the T_1 factor has a range stretching from -1 to $+1$ (depending on the TI and TR values set). This range is twice as large as the maximum range of the SE sequence. This can enhance T_1 contrasts between tissues. In other words: the T_1 weighting in IR images can exceed its influence in SE images. Usually, the IR sequence is used to obtain very strongly T_1 weighted recordings. For this purpose, a TI of about 450 ms must be chosen, while the TR should be at least 1500 ms. The TE is short (18-30 ms), because otherwise there will be too much of a T_2 effect in the images. In this IR sequence, just as in the SE sequence, the T_1 and T_2 effects can counteract each other.

Another advantage of the IR sequence is the possibility of using the *short TI inversion recovery (STIR)* sequence.[44, 45, 61] For this STIR sequence, a very short TI is selected (100-250 ms). Unlike the SE sequence, and the IR sequence normally used (TI = 450 ms), in the STIR sequence, the T_1, T_2 and proton-density effects act in the same direction. For image generation, this means that the influence of the T_1, T_2 and proton-density effects must be added together. Accordingly, tissues with a long T_1, a long T_2, and a high proton density (e.g., tumors and infections) produce a very high signal intensity on the STIR images compared with surrounding tissue. Relatively high tissue contrast is thus obtained. Furthermore, with the help of this sequence, the signal strength of certain tissues can be restricted or even reduced to zero. The latter is the case with a TI of 0.69 times the T_1 value of the tissue concerned. Thus, the signal produced by fat and its effects, for example, can be 'extinguished.' The result of this is

1. improved detection of bone marrow metastases (see also sections 3.3 and 5.3),
2. reduction of respiration artifacts
3. reduction of the 'fat-shift' artifact (see sections 2.5 and 3.3)
4. reduction of interference artifacts arising from the use of surface coils.

A disadvantage of all IR sequences is that the TR must be long enough to allow the protons to readopt their original magnetization state. This results in long imaging times (10-15 min). In general, a TR of three times the T_1 is advised, although in practice it seems that a shorter TR also can be used.

2.3.2.3 *Pulse sequence optimization*

On the basis of formulas similar to the one described in the preceding section, it is possible to estimate the T_1, T_2, and proton-density of certain tissues from a combination of two SE sequences[8] or from a combination of an SE and an IR sequence.[113] Using these data, one can calculate which sequence produces the optimal contrast between tissues. Chapter 3 will describe this in more detail for carcinoma of the urinary bladder.

2.4 Strength of the magnetic field

Currently, medical imaging uses MRI equipment with a field strength of 0.35 to 2.00 Tesla. The stronger the magnetic field, the greater the signal reflected by the body. The signal-to-noise ratio thus increases, resulting in a better quality image at higher field strengths. If the field strength is larger, T_1 is longer.[28] T_2 on the other hand, does not change as a function of the field strength.[81] The fat-shift artifact becomes stronger as the field strength increases (see section 2.5).

2.5 Artifacts

Artifacts often appear during the production of MR images. Many of these artifacts can be reduced or avoided provided their cause is known. This demands knowledge of the design and the mechanism of action of the MR equipment, and also about the method of acquisition, image production and image representation. Some artifacts are clear and disturb the entire image. Others are less clear and only occur in a small part of the image. Some artifacts are unavoidable. It also may be possible to eliminate the artifact reprocessing and/or manipulating the data. Certain artifacts can be very subtle. Some artifacts can be confused with abnormalities.

A number of artifacts that can lead to incorrect interpretation of MR images will be described below. This overview is not complete, but it does deal with the most important artifacts that can arise when imaging the pelvis. For a complete overview of the many MR artifacts, the reader is referred to the literature.[17, 89, 181]

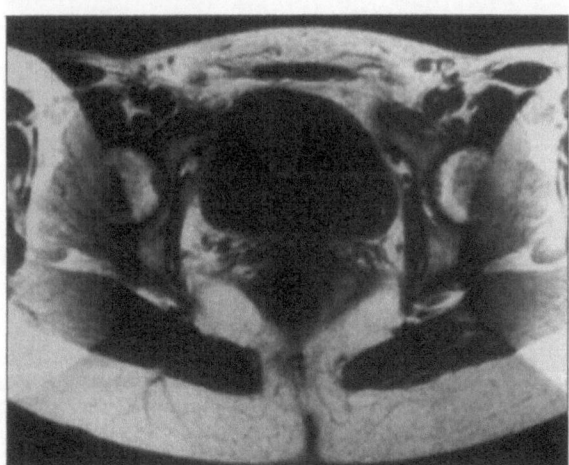

Fig. 2-8. MR image (1.5 T; SE/750/30/4). The 'aliasing' effect can be seen on the sides of the image. In spite of this, the bladder still can be evaluated.

In order to be able to assess artifacts, it is important to recognize the 'direction' in which the artifact occurs. A distinction is made between artifacts occurring in the preparation (phase-encoding) direction and those occurring in the read out (frequency-encoding) direction, perpendicular to the former [129] (see also section 2.2.2).

2.5.1   Aliasing (wraparound) artifact

This artifact occurs if the diameter of the object to be displayed is larger than the field of view. If too small a field is chosen, the outermost part of the image will be projected inward. Provided this inwardly projected part does not superimpose on the areas of diagnostic importance, the image can still be used (Fig. 2-8). The artifact is visible in the direction of preparation. To avoid these effects, one can
1. interchange the preparation and the readout directions,
2. enlarge the field of view,
3. use a filter, or
4. use surface coils, which prevent any signal from being received from the 'interfering' tissue.

2.5.2   Fat-shift artifact

These artifacts occur because the proton spins in water and fat have a slightly different resonant frequency. This results in a dark or light signal on the boundary areas of water and fat. The fat shift artifact can be seen in the frequency-encoding (readout)

direction.[17] Considering the bladder wall forms the boundary of strongly bound (fat) and less strongly bound protons (water in smooth muscle tissue), part of this wall may be less easy to assess because of the fat shift artifact. Black and white artifact lines can, therefore, be seen precisely at the site of the thin bladder wall (Figs. 2-9 and 2-10). This artifact can be reduced by:
1. lowering the field strength of the magnetic field: the fat shift (expressed in Hertz) is directly proportional to the field strength (Fig. 2-9). However, as the field strength decreases, the general image quality also will decrease (see section 2.4),
2. interchanging the 'readout' and 'preparation' directions. In this way, the entire bladder can be easily assessed (Fig.2-10),
3. making the readout gradient steeper,
4. making use of a certain recording technique that produces a 'fat' and 'water' image. These images can then be combined into an image free of chemical artifact.

2.5.3   Artifacts caused by patients' movement

These artifacts can be recognized as:
1. Vague double images ('ghost artifacts'). These occur in the preparation direction (Fig.2-10) and are independent of the direction in which the movement occurs. The artifacts become more pronounced with an increase in TR or movement.
2. A blurring of the image. This blurring occurs in the direction of movement (e.g., intestinal move-

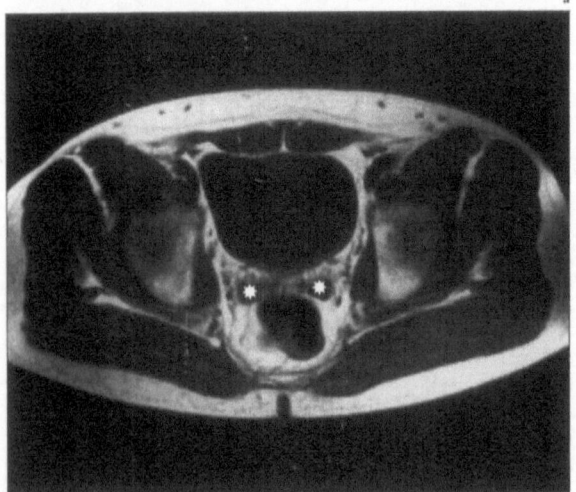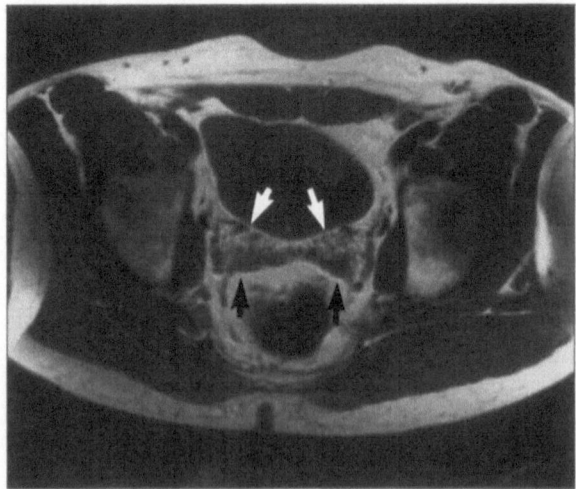

Fig. 2-9. (a) The MR image (0.5 T; SE/750/30/4) shows hardly any fat-shift artifact. **(b)** On the MR image made at 1.5 T with identical parameters, a fat-shift artifact causes interference in the ventrodorsal direction (see arrows). The seminal vesicles (*) have a symmetrical intermediate signal intensity.

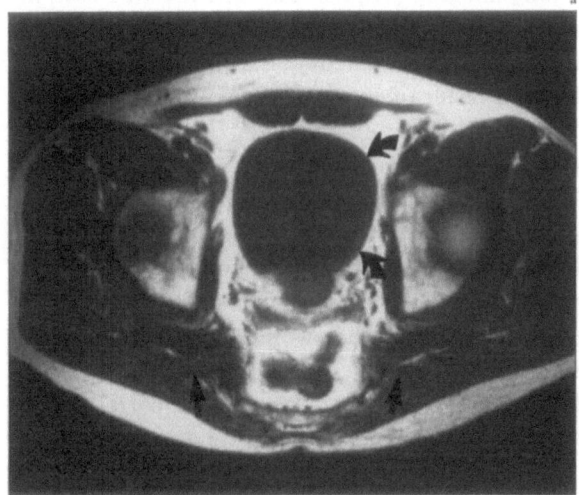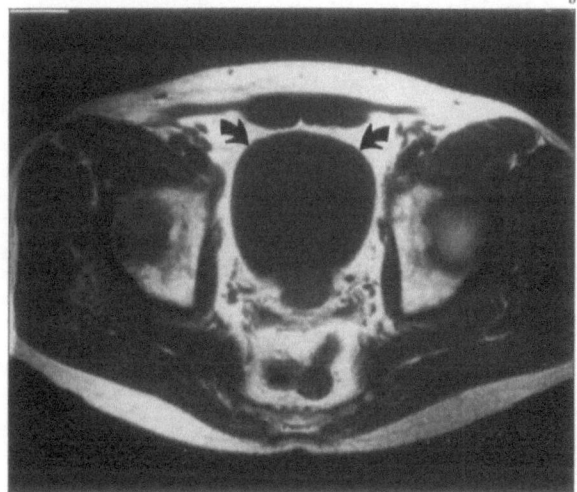

Fig. 2-10. MR images with identical parameters (1.5 T; SE/750/30/2). **(a)** With ventrodorsal preparation direction, the fat-shift artifact (curved arrows) can be seen in the left-right and the motion artifacts (straight arrows) in the ventrodorsal direction; **(b)** With a left-right preparation direction, the fat-shift artifact is in the ventrodorsal direction. The motion artifacts in the left-right direction can hardly be seen.

ment, or movement due to respiration). Section 3.2 discusses how motion artifacts can be reduced.

2.5.4   Metal artifacts

Ferromagnetic or partly ferromagnetic objects cause artifacts because they have a greater affinity for the magnetic field than do the surrounding tissues.[125] This results in distortion of the image and alteration in contrast.[73, 133, 141] The direction of the incorrect image registration depends on the readout gradient. The characteristic image is that of an area with a very low or completely absent signal intensity, surrounded by an area of increased signal intensity. Serious distortion of the image often occurs (Fig. 2-11). This distortion can be so bad that the image is no longer usable.

The size of the artifact is determined by the degree of ferromagnetism of the material causing this artifact. Ferromagnetic material is present in surgical suture material (e.g., sternal sutures), surgical clips, prosthesis (e.g., hip prosthesis), zippers, safety pins, jewelry (not made of gold or silver), and mascara.

When generating an image of the bladder, surgical clips (often placed on lymphatic vessels after lymphadenectomy) and hip prostheses are important. The artifacts caused by these do not interfere with imaging of the bladder. The stripe artifacts that these

materials produce on CT scans are much more troublesome (Fig. 2-12). The urinary bladder cannot be assessed on a CT scan of a patient with a total hip prosthesis, but it can be assessed on an MR image.[141]

2.6   Advantages of MRI over other imaging techniques

Creating images of parts of the human body by means of MRI can be achieved non invasively. MRI does not bother the patient very much and there are no known side effects. Unlike other imaging techniques, MRI seems to offer an almost unlimited number of possibilities for intensifying the contrast between tissues. In addition to generating an image that reflects the distribution of proton density, information also can be obtained about the mutual interaction and coherence of the protons (see section 2.2). On the basis of T_1 and T_2 times, this results in improved differentiation between certain tissues.

Another advantage of MRI is the possibility of obtaining an image in any plane at any slice thickness or slice interval. With MRI, blood vessels can be displayed without having to administer contrast agents.[12] Thus, lymph nodes can easily be distinguished from blood vessels (Fig. 2-13). Also, dynamic information can be obtained about the flow through vascular structures.

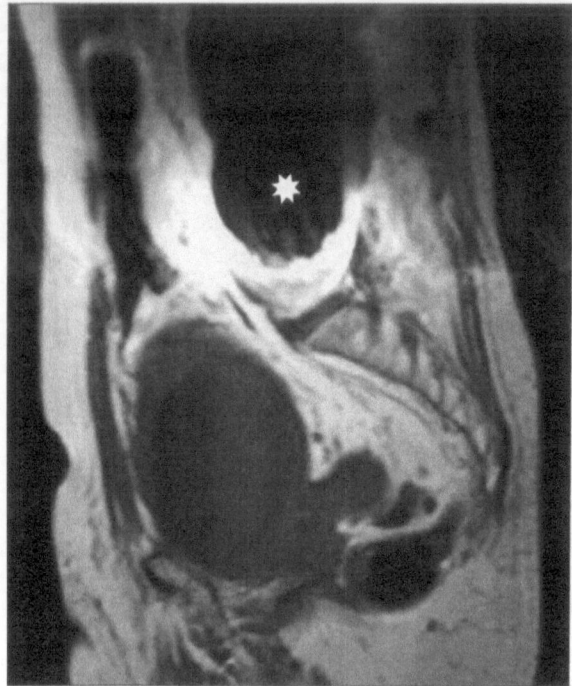

Fig. 2-11. MR image (1.5 T; SE/800/30/2) shows distorsion and areas of increased and decreased (*) signal intensity where a metal guide wire was left behind after a nephrostomy.

Finally, MRI offers the potential, in combination with MRS, to acquire more quantitative information about physiological and biochemical processes of certain tissue structures in the body.

2.7 Disadvantages of MRI compared with other imaging techniques

In addition to its advantages, MRI also has a few disadvantages compared with other techniques.

A long imaging (acquisition) time must be used in order to obtain a good quality image (high signal-to-noise ratio). This can reduce the quality of the image due as a result of *motion artifacts*. The acquistion time varies from a few minutes (for a T_1 weighted image) to tens of minutes (for a T_2 weighted image). Sequences are being developed, however, that allow a considerably shorter acquisition time. These include: fast field echo (FFE), fast imaging with steady precession (FISP), fast low angle shot (FLASH) and gradient refocussed acquisition in the steady state (GRASS) sequences (see section 6.2.3). Also, nowadays, images can be made that can be corrected for breathing movements and heart action.

Approximately 1-5% of all patients suffer from *claustrophobia* because of lying for such a long time in the narrow tunnel of the MR scanners. Sedatives and anxiolytics can help, as can having the patient lie prone.

The *high cost* of an MRI examination ($ 500)[192] is the biggest disadvantage. The equipment must be installed according to certain rules. It must be magnetically isolated from the environment, which entails considerable (and hence costly) requirements with regard to installation.

Evaluation of the diagnostic benefit, and the accompanying benefits of a more specific choice of therapy and reduction of other examinations (which may be expensive and not always without risk to the patient) is, therefore, certainly desirable. Expensive examinations include angiography, skeletal scintigraphy, and

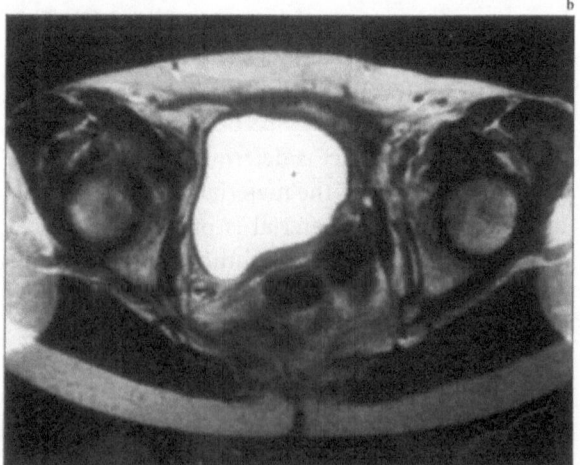

Fig. 2-12. (a) Metal clips cause stripe artifacts on CT scan. **(b)** On the MR image (1.5 T; SE/800/30/4) (after Gd-DTPA), no artifacts can be seen.

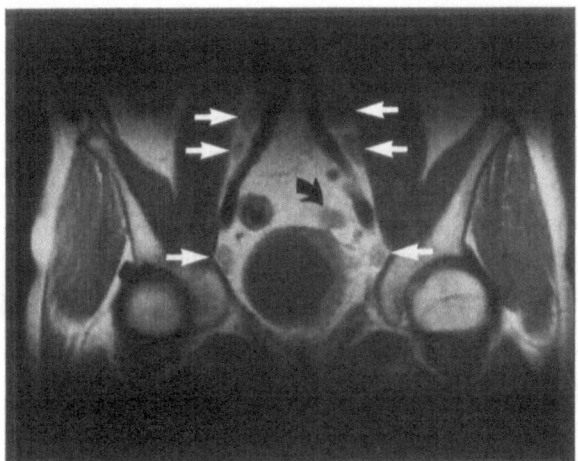

Fig. 2-13. On the coronal MR image (0.5 T; SE/2000/30/2), the gray abnormally enlarged lymph nodes (arrows) can easily be distinguished from the low-signal iliac arteries. It is difficult to differentiate between intestine (curved arrow) and lymph node.

CT. Studies that involve some risk or are troublesome for the patient include angiography, lymphography, and CT with contrast injection.

2.8 Safety of MRI

This section examines the possible dangers of MRI that can arise from physical and physiological effects.[235] These effects can be subdivided into short-term and long-term effects.

2.8.1 Short-term effects

These effects can be divided into three categories:
1. effects resulting from the static magnetic field,
2. effects resulting from electrical currents, induced by the main magnetic field varying in time, and
3. effects resulting from heat generated by the RF signal.

2.8.1.1 Static magnetic field

There are eight effects known to result from the static magnetic field:
a. attraction by the magnetic field of ferromagnetic objects outside the patient,
b. traction on ferromagnetic objects inside the patient,
c. interference with pacemakers,
d. changes in enzyme kinetics,[40, 168, 182]
e. magnetohemodynamic interactions,[39]
f. electrical current induction in the cardiovascular system,[40]
g. effects on the speed of conduction in nerves,[82, 144]
h. changes in orientation of molecules and cell structures.[40, 83, 160, 163]

The last five effects do not occur under the valid norms for use of MRI apparatus, nor do they play a part in the clinical use of MRI. Those interested in the last five effects are referred to the references cited.

Attraction of ferromagnetic objects outside the patient

Ferromagnetic objects are attracted by the magnetic field, and this can cause metal objects to fly into the magnet just like projectiles. An extra danger can arise if these objects line up parallel to the axis of the magnetic field. Sharp objects such as scissors and knives will thus fly through the magnetic tunnel with the point at the front or back and penetrate anything in their way. To date, no serious accidents have been reported, because the rules concerning entering the scanning room are very strict.

As current resuscitation equipment is extremely ferromagnetic, in the case of a cardiovascular emergency, the patient would have to be removed from the scanning room. Nor is it possible to artificially respirate a patient an scanner. The development of non ferromagnetic respiratory equipment is being investigated as a way of overcoming this limitation.

Traction on ferromagnetic implants

As a result of the magnetic field, forces are exerted on ferromagnetic implants. This can lead to traction on the implant or to torsion. These forces can be considerable. New et al.[166] described an experiment in which two aneurysm clips on the femoral artery of a rat were exposed to a 1.47-T magnetic field. Considerable rotation ensued, which, however, did not result in the vessel being torn loose.
The risk of traction and torsion depends on
- the strength and the gradient of the magnetic field,
- the magnetization component of the ferromagnetic implant

- the mass, form, and degree of ferromagnetism of the implant (this dependens on the alloy and, unfortunately, is often unknown),
- the anatomic location of the implant,
- the fixation of the implant to the surrounding structures, and finally
- the vulnerability of the tissues to which the implant is attached.

A metal implant with a slight ferromagnetic effect will hardly reveal any traction or torsion during an MRI examination.[73] Metal implants with a strong ferromagnetism do, however, show a large degree of displacement during MRI examinations. Accordingly, patients with strong ferromagnetic implants cannot undergo MRI. Thus, it is very important to determine the degree of ferromagnetism of implants before the MRI examination. The effects on aortic valve prostheses are not important clinically (except for the old Starr-Edwards heart valve prosthesis). Patients with valve prostheses can, therefore, undergo examination without appreciable risk.[210] Orthopedic implants (e.g., total hip prostheses and Harrington's rods) do not pose a problem.[141]

Interference with pacemakers

A field strength of more than 17 mT can influence the rhythm of a pacemaker.

2.8.1.2 *Effects of electrical currents induced by the main magnetic field varying in time*

According to Faraday's laws of induction, a magnetic field varying in time gives rise to an electric current. There are three known effects on the human body:[39]

a. stimulation of visual flash sensations,[7, 38, 40, 41]
b. stimulation of nerves and induction of heart fibrillation,[38, 40, 133, 173, 190] and
c. a positive effect on bone healing. [15, 40]

These effects are not significant for the current norms established by the Food and Drug Administration (USA).

2.8.1.3 *Warming/heating effect of RF signals*

The fast change in RF field induces currents, which produce warmth in the body as a result of the resistance that they encounter. Most of the heat will develop on the surface, so that the maximum increase in temperature can be expected in the skin and the subcutaneous fat. Not all RF energy is absorbed by the body: 60% of all energy is reflected by the boundary between tissue and air. Another part passes through the body without any interaction. Recent investigations have shown that the maximal energy absorption allowed (4 W/kg) can be reasonably well tolerated even by older patients with poor cardiovascular function and possible interaction of medication and thermoregulation. After a recording time of 20 min, a maximal increase in skin temperature of 1°C was measured.[2, 40]

Absorption of RF energy by large metal implants can lead to a significant increase in temperature, especially if the blood circulation is restricted.[52] During normal MRI examinations, however, no side effects have been described in patients with metal prostheses.[133, 141, 156] Nor are significant increases in temperature measured in heart valves or hip prostheses.[37, 210]

2.8.2   Long-term effects:

To date, there are no known disadvantageous long-term effects of MRI. NMR investigations with strong magnetic fields have been being performed in biochemistry since 1948. As yet, no side effect has been reported by people working with these magnets.[173] Long-term exposure to MR pulse sequences has not caused any demonstrable genetic or cytogenetic damage,[232] nor is there evidence of behavioral disturbances or loss of memory in rats exposed for long periods to MR.[231].

No damaging effects are known to result from exposure to MR during the first trimester of pregnancy, either in the mother or in the fetus. Specifically, induction of congenital abnormalities in the fetus has not been reported.[96]

Currently, the greatest risk of MRI lies in incorrect or incomplete interpretation of the images, as a result of limited experience with the technique.[3]

In summary: the potential dangers of MRI lurk mainly in the effects of the strong static magnetic field. The following factors are important:

- direct mechanical effect on ferromagnetic objects, which thus fly to the magnet and can injure the patient,

- movement, such as turning of ferromagnetic implants (especially vessel clips), and
- interference with pacemakers.

Other effects cause no danger to the patient, provided the field strength, the speed of change of the magnetic field and the RF energy do exceed the set limits.[165] Studies have shown that these limits are safe and fixed with a wide margin. One would expect that these limits will be raised as experience with MRI increases.

2.9 Contraindications for MRI investigation

The contraindications for MRI can be deduced from the preceding sections. The following are currently considered to be contraindications for an MRI examination:

1. patients with a *pacemaker,*
2. patients with *ferromagnetic vessel clips,* and
3. patients with *the old Starr-Edwards heart-valve prosthesis;*
4. although there are no known teratogenic effects in humans,[96] for reasons of safety it is advised that no MRI examination be performed during *the first 3 months of pregnancy;*[128]
5. finally, *patients with claustrophobia* will exclude themselves from an MRI examination; should it prove absolutely necessary, MRI can be performed in these patients if they are given anxiolytics or sedatives.

III

TECHNICAL ASPECTS OF MRI SPECIFIC RELEVANT TO PATIENTS WITH CARCINOMA OF THE URINARY BLADDER.

3.1 Introduction, optimal conditions for examination

This chapter attempts to give describe which conditions result in optimal MR images of the urinary bladder, of the UBC, and of the metastases of UBC (in particular lymph node and bone marrow metastases). These factors can be divided into four groups.

First of all it is important to minimize the *patient-related factors* as much as possible. Motion artifacts and the degree to which the bladder is distended are relevant here.

Second, as already described in Chapter 2, certain sequences lead to optimal contrast in the MR image. There must be a good degree of contrast between the UBC and the surrounding structures so that it can be discriminated. This *optimization of the pulse sequence* will be described in section 3.3.

Third, *surface coils* can improve the quality of the image. The value of these coils in staging of the UBC will be evaluated in section 3.4.

Finally, section 3.5 will deal with the effect of *magnetic field strenght* (0.5 and 1.5 Tesla) on imaging of UBC.

3.2 Patient-related factors

A number of patient-related factors are important for good MR imaging. The most important are motion artifacts and degree of bladder distension.

Movement artifacts have already been described in section 2.5. They can be voluntary or involuntary, and possible means of reducing them are described in the following sections.

3.2.1 Voluntary motion artifacts

First of all, these artifacts can be reduced by making the patient feel at ease. It is essential to explain the procedure fully before starting the examination. Sedation can be administered if the patient is very tense.

Voluntary motion artifacts also can be reduced by using as short a scanning time as possible, for example by using 'fast' sequences (see section 6.2.3) or by diminishing the 'phase-encoding' (preparation) axis (e.g., a 128 x 256 rather than a 256 x 256 matrix).

3.2.2 Involuntary motion artifacts

These are caused by cardiac motion, respiration, intestinal peristalsis, and bladder motions. The motions artifacts resulting from *cardiac motion* are not relevant when imaging the pelvis.

Respiration, intestinal peristalsis, and bladder motions can have a negative effect on the production of an MR image of the true pelvis. In order to reduce respiratory motions, a tight band can be wrapped around the upper abdomen of the patient. The disturbing movements of intestine and bladder can be counteracted by giving the patient 0.5 ml Buscopan intravenously and 1.5 ml intramuscularly immediately before to the first sequence. Another way of minimizing these motion artifacts is to ensure that the patient does not take anything orally for 4 hours before the examination.[229] Respiratory motions can also be corrected by using the so-called 'respiratory gating' technique or by altering the preparation direction by an angle of 90. In the latter case, the motion artifacts turn up at a different location where they do not interfere with the imaging process. Moreover, the use of new 'fast' sequences (see section 6.2.3) is found to be very promising here. With these sequences, the recording time can be shortened, and this considerably reduces motion artifacts.

3.2.3 Bladder distension

Optimal bladder distension is very important. A bladder that is not sufficiently distended results in contraction of the detrusor muscle. The thickening of this muscle layer makes it very difficult to recognise small abnormalities (Fig. 3-1). If the bladder becomes too full, the patient becomes restless and flat tumors can be missed because of the muscle layer being overstretched (Fig. 3-2).

Thus, for optimal imaging, the bladder should be reasonably well filled. In general, this can be achieved by asking the patient to urinate 2 hours before the examination and then not again until the examination is completed.

3.3 Pulse-sequence optimization

As described in Chapter 2, certain sequences will produce an optimal image contrast between certain tissues and organs. This optimal contrast is necessary to differentiate these structures. The optimal sequences for MRI of UBC and how these can be

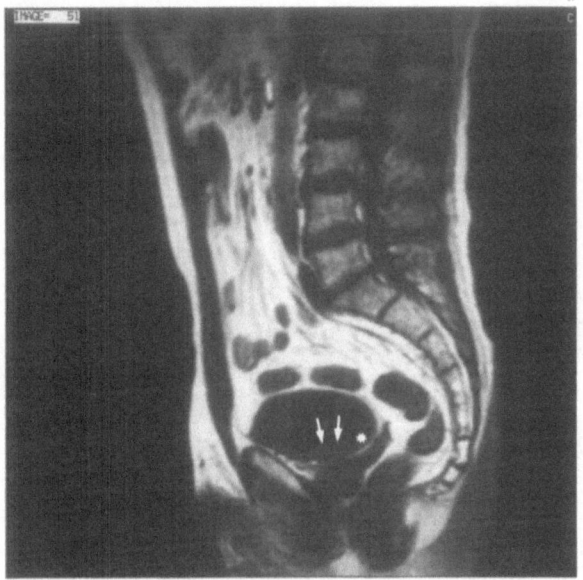 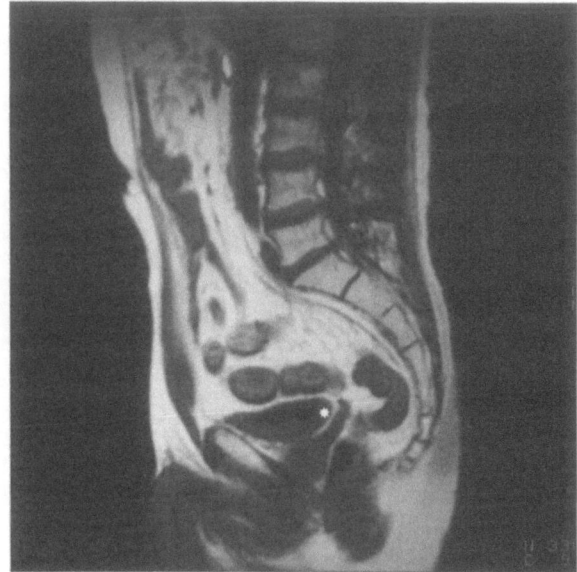

Fig. 3-1. (a) On the MR image (1.5 T; SE/750/30/2), a tumor is visible on the floor of the urinary bladder (arrows). (b) This tumor cannot be distinguished on the MR image made with the patient's bladder empty (identical patient positioning and parameters) because of contraction of the detrusor muscle.
* = plica interureterica.

determined will be explained in the following paragraphs.

First of all, the sequences described in the literature are reviewed. Then the value of these sequences in patients with UBC is assessed. After this, two methods for determining the optimal sequences are described. Finally, an indication is given of which sequences can best be used to generate an image of UBC, taking into account the possibilities offered by the MR scanner and the patient.

3.3.1 Literature review

When diagnosing UBC, it is important to be able to differentiate:
a. the tumor from the perivesical fat and nearby organs,
b. the tumor from the normal bladder wall,
c. the tumor from the urine in the bladder,
d. pathologic lymph nodes (i.e. tumor) from normal lymph nodes and from the retroperitoneal and parailiac fat and finally,
e. bone marrow metastases (tumor) from normal bone marrow (fat).

Between the bladder and the surrounding organs there is usually a thin layer of fat. An exception to

this is the prostate (see also Chapter 4). Tumour invasion of nearby organs can be determined on the basis of whether or not this thin fat layer is present. If it has disappeared, then tumor invasion is probable. Hence, in order to determine invasion of surrounding organs, it is very important to be able to distinguish between fat and tumor. This is also the case when determining the presence of lymph node and bone marrow metastases. After all, lymph nodes are surrounded by fat, and bone marrow also contains mainly fat (see also Chapter 4).

Therefore, to determine tumor invasion of perivesical fat and nearby organs (except the prostate) and to establish lymph node and bone marrow metastases, it is important to have optimal distinction between *tumor and fat*.

When assessing tumor invasion of the prostate, one must not only look at invasion of the tumor into the prostate itself, but one also should be aware of the possibility of invasion into the thin layer of bladder muscle that lies on top of it. Optimal contrast between *tumor and bladder wall* (muscle layer) is important here.

Finally, it is important, when assessing the shape of the tumor (papillary or flat), to be able to differentiate *tumor from urine*.

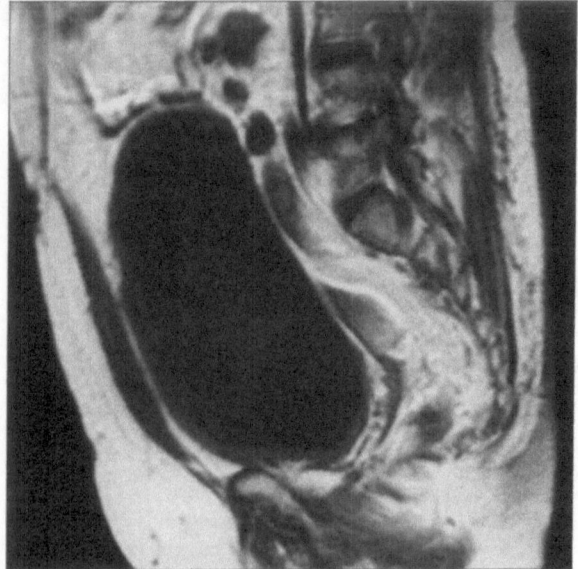 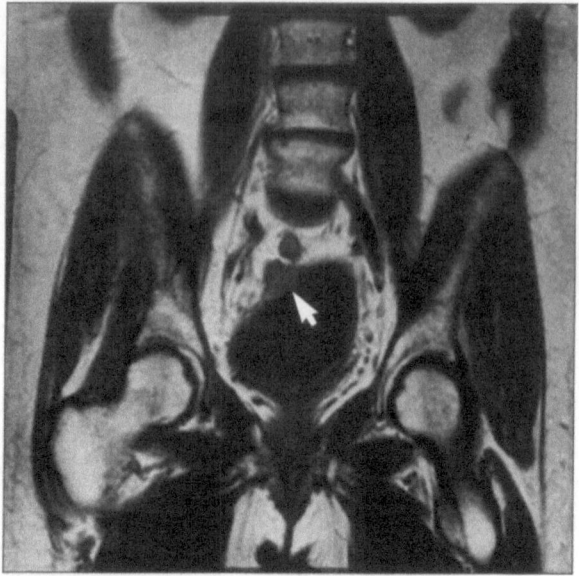

Fig. 3-2. (a) A flat tumor cannot be seen on the sagittal MR image (1.5 T; SE/800/30/2) because the patients bladder is too full. **(b)** On the coronal image, made when the patients bladder was not so full, the tumor can be detected (arrow).

For the diagnosis of UBC, the literature reports the use of both T_1- and T_2-weighted images. A survey of the sequences used is presented in Table 9.

The authors in this table indicate that the greatest contrast between fat and tumor is obtained with T_1-weighted SE sequences. For this purpose, the SE/400-800/21-35 sequences are used (sequence type/TR/TE). With these T_1-weighted sequences, the image quality is good and the imaging time is short (5 min).

T_2-weighted SE sequences (i.e. the SE/1600-2100/-56-240 sequences) are recommended for differentiation of tumor from bladder wall (prostate) and tumor from urine. Here, the TE is on average 100 ms. It is quite feasible to distinguish between tumor and urine on both T_1- and T_2-weighted SE-images.

It should be pointed out that these authors used different field strengths (0.35-1.5 T). As described in section 2.4, T_1 increases with field strength,[28] while T_2 is independent of it. MR images made at higher field strengths have a less strong T_1 effect at the same sequence parameters. Consequently, the T_1-weighted MR images made at higher field strength are less T_1- weighted than images made at lower field strength, and T_2 weighted images made at hig-

her field strenght are more T_2 weighted. It is noticeable that in spite of the difference in field strength, the 'ideal' sequences described in Table 9 do not differ very much.

Only two authors[76, 126] calculated T_1, T_2, and proton- density values for tumor, urine, bladder wall and fat on the basis of a combination of two SE sequences (method according to Feinberg et al.[70]). Koelbel et al.[126] did this in 7 patients, Fisher et al.[76] in 30. Unfortunately, the values found were not used to calculate the optimal sequence. Three other authors did determine the optimal sequence parameters for fat-tumor, tumor- urine, and tumor-bladder wall differentiation by means of contrast measurements for 4, 10 and 8 combinations, respectively, of TE and TR.[76,126,131] Here, Fisher et al. used a field strength of 0.35 T, Koelbel et al. and Küper et al. used 1.5 T. These authors found the ideal sequence for differentiation of tumor from fat to be SE/500/28, SE/400-600/30 and SE/800/30 respectively.

According to Fisher et al., the optimal sequence for differentiation between tumor and bladder wall was SE/2000/60, according to Küper et al. SE/1600/30, and according to Koelbel et al. SE/2000/240. Three remarks must be made at this point.

First of all, the longest TE used by Fisher et al. [76]

was 56 ms. Second, Küper et al. [131] did not investigate the SE/2000/90 sequence. Third, Koelbel et al. [126] did not report the quality of the image made with their SE/2000/240 sequence.

Hence, there was no question of structured or systematic pulse-sequence optimization for UBC. Nevertheless, there is still considerable agreement on the pulse sequences to use.

3.3.2 Evaluation of sequences most frequently used in the literature

When the present study was initiated, it was not feasible to determine the optimal pulse sequence, so the most frequently used sequences were adopted from the published data described in the preceding section. In addition, the sequences used were limited by the MR equipment available. In this study, the value of these sequences was evaluated in 142 patients with UBC. The composition of this group of patients will be described in Chapter 5.

At the start of the study, a magnetic field strength of 0.5 T was used to perform 41 MRI examinations in 37 patients with a UBC. In 1987, the field strength was converted to 1.5 T. One hundred thirty-one MRI examinations were performed in 105 patients with UBC.

The sequences used at 0.5 T were SE/400-800/30/2 (41 times), (sequence type/TR/TE/number of excitations), SE/2000/30,60/2 (12 times), SE/2000/30,100/2 (17 times), and SE/2000/30,150/2 (8 times).

At 1.5 T the sequenced used were SE/400-800/30/2 (131 times), SE/2000/30,100/2 (100 times), SE/2000/30,150/2 (8 times), and SE/3000/30,100/1 (7 times).

On the basis of promising results with the STIR sequence (see also section 2.3.2.2), the IR/2000/100/30,60/2 sequence (sequence type/TR/TI/TE/number of excitations) also was used in 12 patients.

3.3.2.1 T_1-weighted sequences

At 0.5 T, the image quality was mediocre in 2 of the 41 examinations, in 2 it was reasonable, in 36 it was good and in 1 very good. At 1.5 T, the quality of the image was poor in 1 of the 131 MRI examinations, mediocre in 9, reasonable in 21, good in 90 and very good in 10. The poor and mediocre quality of images was due to motion artifacts.

The signal-to-noise ratio was high, and this produced a good quality image. The contrast between

Table 9 Survey of pulse sequences used in published reports.

		field strength (in T)	T_1-weighted sequence (TR/TE)	T_2-weighted sequence (TR/TE)
Lenz et al.	(1985) [142]	0,5	400/35	1600/35 + 70
Buy et al.	(1988) [43]	0,5	400/28	1600/40 + 80 + 120
Nicolas et al.	(1988) [167]	0,5 – 1,5	500/21 – 30	1800/50 + 150
Fisher et al.	(1985) [76]	0,35	500/28	2000/28 + 56
Amendola et al.	(1986) [6]	0,35	500/28	2000/56
Rholl et al.	(1987) [188]	0,35 – 0,5	500/30 – 35	2100/30 + 90
Küper et al.	(1986) [131]	1,5	600/30	1600/30 + 150
Koebel et al.	(1988) [126]	1,5	800/30	2000/90 + 240
Beyer et al.	(1985) [20]	0,35	400/35	1600/35 + 120
Bryan et al.	(1987) [35]	0,35 – 1,0	500/30 – 50	2000/35 + 75 – 90
Lee et al.	(1986) [139]	0,5	500/30	2100/90 + 120
		0,35 – 1,5	400 – 800/ 21 – 35	1600 – 2100/ 30 – 35 + 56 – 240

tumor and fat and between bladder wall and fat was excellent.

Tumour and bladder wall appeared gray on the image, while the perivesical fat was white (Fig. 3-3). There was no difference in signal between tumor and bladder wall. The contrast between tumor and urine and bladder wall and urine was reasonable, enabling demarcation of the intravesicular part of the tumor and the bladder wall. In this situation, tumor and bladder wall were gray and the urine was dark (Fig. 3-3).

With identical sequence parameters, the contrast between tumor and urine and between bladder wall and urine at 0.5 T was slightly better than at 1.5 T.

3.3.2.2 T_2-weighted sequences

In 37 patients with carcinoma of the urinary bladder, 41 T_2- weighted images were produced at a field strength of 0.5 T. At a field strength of 1.5 T, 119 T_2-weighted images were produced in 105 patients. Eight sequences could not be assessed because of motion artifacts (four at 0.5 T and four at 1.5 T).
In all of these images made with T_2-weighted sequences, an evaluation was made of how the signal

intensity of a local thickening of the bladder wall (visible on the T_1-weighted images) compared with that of the normal bladder wall. This local thickening correlated with the place where a tumor was observed during cystoscopy.

The signal intensity of this thickening was scored as 'higher' than or 'equal' to that of the normal bladder wall. 'Higher' meant that the thickening definitely had a higher signal intensity than the normal bladder wall. 'Equal' indicated an equal signal intensity.
Within 4 weeks of the MRI examination, the histologic diagnosis of wall thickening was achieved by cystectomy (40 patients) or by transurethral resection (remaining patients) in all patients. If no UBC was found histologically, this was scored as T0. In these cases, histologic examination of the wall thickening revealed fibrous and granular tissue. If histologic study revealed UBC, this was scored as T+.

In addition to being aware of contrast between tumor and bladder wall on MR images, attention was also paid to contrast between bladder wall and urine and between tumor and urine. Table 10A and 10B present a survey of the T_2-weighted sequences used, the contrast between wall thickening (tumor) and bladder wall, and the histologic findings.

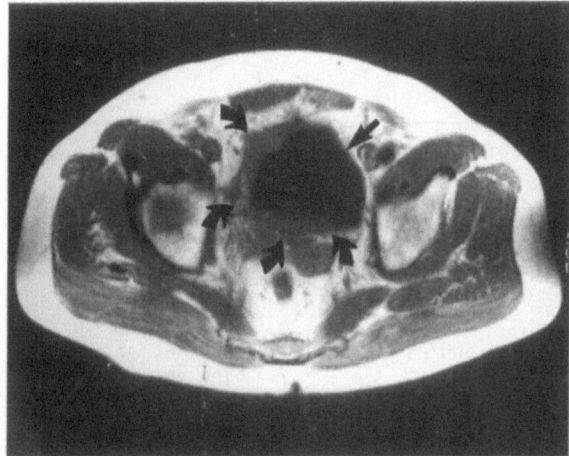

Fig. 3-3. On the T1-weighted MR image (0.5 T; SE/750/30/2), the tumor (curved arrows) and the normal bladder wall (arrow) appear gray. The latter is, however, very thin. The extension of the tumor into the white perivesical fat can be assessed well. The intravesicular part of the tumor also can be easily distinguished from the dark urine.

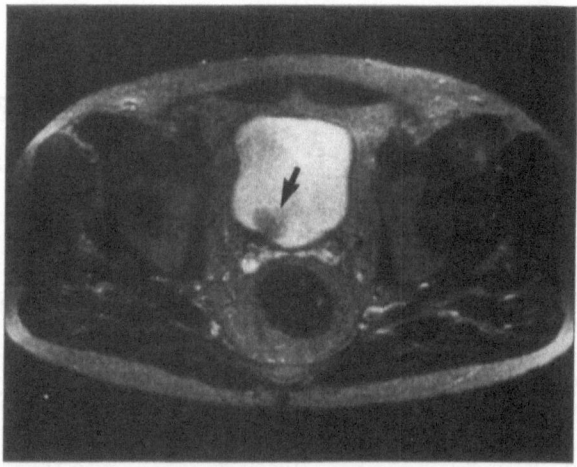

Fig. 3-4. Strongly T2-weighted MR image (0.5 T; SE/2000/150/2). The papillar tumor (arrow) clearly has a higher signal intensity than the dark bladder wall. Bladder wall and tumor can be easily distinguished on this image from the white urine. The bladder wall is not interrupted at the site of the tumor, which indicates that invasion into the muscle layer is not deep (stage Ta-T2).

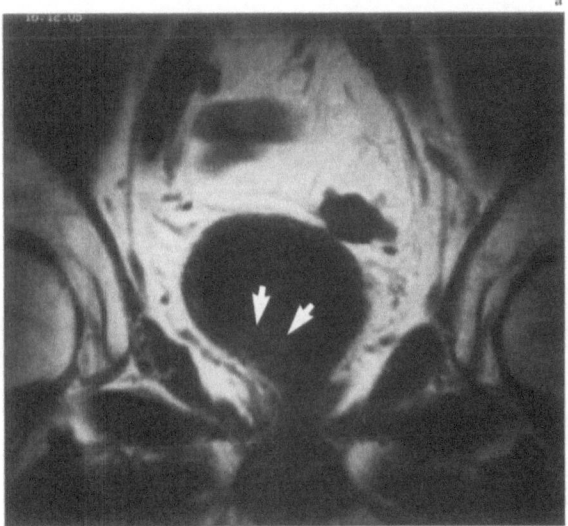 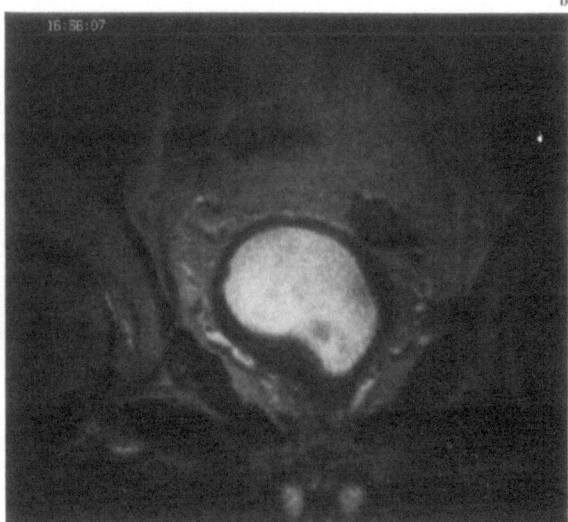

Fig. 3-5. (a) Local thickening of the bladder wall can be seen (arrows) on the T1-weighted coronal MR image (1.5 T; SE/750/15/2). **(b)** On the T2-weighted image (1.5 T; SE/2000/100/2), this thickening has just as low a signal intensity as the bladder wall, indicating fibrosis. This was confirmed histologically.

0.5 Tesla:

In accordance with what one would expect on the basis of published data (all authors in Table 7), the signal intensity of UBC was, in general, higher than that of the bladder wall (Fig. 3-4). Fibrous and granular tissue, on the other hand, produced an equal, low signal intensity (Fig. 3-5).

The impression was that the results obtained with the SE/2000/60/2 sequence were the best. A disadvantage of this sequence was, however, difficulty in distinguishing between malignant tissue and urine (Fig. 3-6).

On all T2-weighted images with a very long TE (100 or 150 ms), the contrast between bladder wall and urine and between tumor and urine was sufficiently great to allow them to be differentiated from each other. Thus, these sequences were preferred. Thus, the findings with a TE of 150 ms were slightly more favourable.

1.5 Tesla:

UBC also gave a clearly higher signal intensity than the bladder wall at a magnetic field strength of 1.5 T on the T2- weighted images: for the SE/2000/100/2, SE/2000/150/2, and SE/3000/100/1 sequences, the percentages of patients in whom UBC had a higher signal intensity the bladder wall were 86%, 63% and 83% respectively.

In seven patients, a higher signal intensity was found at the site of the wall thickening, which did *not*

appear to be the result of UBC (Fig. 3-7). In addition to fibrous and granular tissue, infected tissue also was present. The latter was probably the cause of the increased signal intensity. Other authors also have reported difficulty in differentiating between malignant infiltration and benign infection.[76,126]

In 13 patients, no difference in signal could be found between malignant tumor and bladder wall. A possible explanation for this is a raised signal intensity of the bladder wall caused by infection (e.g., due to chronic cystitis or chemotherapy or radiotherapy).

Because of the long TE, the signal-to-noise ratio of the SE/2000/150/2 sequence was mediocre. The signal-to-noise ratio with the same sequence at a field strength of 0.5 T could be improved by using a 'double surface coil' (see section 3.4). The signal-to-noise ratio of the SE/3000/100/1 sequence also was mediocre because only one measurement was used. This could not be avoided as the imaging time at this TR for two measurements would (otherwise) be too long.

Differentiation between tumor and urine was quite possible at a field strength of 1.5 T with all T2-weighted sequences.

STIR-sequence (see also section 2.3.2.2)

The STIR sequence chosen was that described in the literature: IR/2000/120/30,60/2.[44, 45, 61] With this sequence, structures with long T_1 and long T_2 (e.g.,

Table 10 A   Signal intensity of wall thickening compared with that of normal urinary bladder wall on T_2 weighted images with histologic diagnosis (0,5 T).

		contrast of wall thickening compared with that of bladder wall		
		higher	equal	number of patients
Sequence:				
SE/2000/100/2:	T0:	1	**3**	4
	T+:	**10**	3	13
				17
SE/2000/150/2:	T0:	0	1	1
	T+:	6	1	7
				8
SE/2000/60/2:	T0:	0	**2**	2
	T+:	**10**	0	10
				12
			Total	37

Table 10 B   Signal intensity of wall thickening compared with that of normal urinary bladder wall on T_2 weighted images with histologic diagnosis (1,5 T).

		contrast of wall thickening compared with that of bladder wall		
		higher	equal	number of patients
Sequence:				
SE/2000/100/2:	T0:	7	**22**	29
	T+:	**61**	10	71
				100
SE/2000/150/2:	T0:	0	1	1
	T+:	6	1	7
				8
SE/3000/100/1:	T0:	0	1	1
	T+:	5	1	6
				7
			Total	115

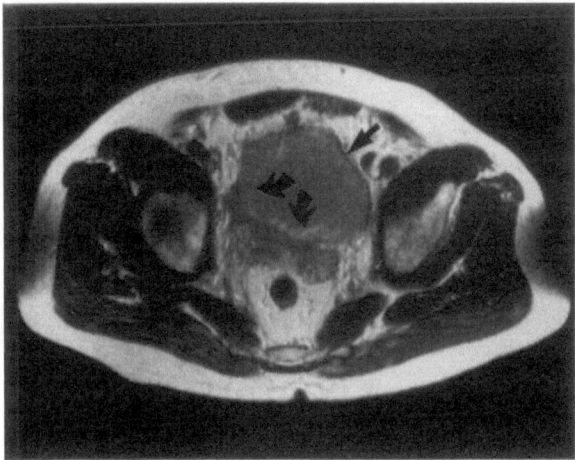

Fig. 3-6. Transverse MR image (SE/2000/60/2). Most of the bladder wall has been infiltrated by tumor. There is still a thin layer of normal wall on the left side (straight arrow). The signal intensities of tumor and urine are equal. A thin layer of higher signal intensity covers the tumor (curved arrows); this is compatible with mucosal inflammation.

3.3.2.3 *Proton-weighted sequences*

Without extending the acquisition time, it was possible to obtain images with a shorter TE at the same time as the T₂-weighted images.

In order to obtain information about the effect of proton density on MR images, a TE of 30 ms was selected on the basis of published data (Table 9). With this sequence (SE/2000/30/2), MR images were obtained in which the T_1 and T_2 effects were equally strong. Considering that these effects in the SE sequence counteracted each other with regard to signal intensity, an image was produced that contained a great deal of information about proton density. On these images, inflammation of the mucous membrane layer of the urinary bladder was clearly visible (see Fig. 4-2 and 4-5a).

3.3.3 Determination of the optimal pulse sequence (1.5 T)

Halfway through the study described here, it became possible to produce an image based on a combination of an SE sequence and an IR sequence, from which the T_1 and T_2 values of various tissues and organs could be determined.

On the basis of these values, 'contrast matrices' were constructed, from which the sequences with optimal contrast between tumor and fat, tumor and bladder wall and tumor and urine could be derived. The results of these optimal sequences in 14 patients with UBC will be discussed in sections 3.3.3.1 and 3.3.3.2.

tumor, infection, and urine) could easily be recognized by their very high signal intensity (Fig. 3-8). The fat signal also could be eliminated (Fig. 3-9).

The fat-shift artifact between the perivesical fat and the bladder wall was minimal. Motion artifacts caused by fat were less disturbing than on T₂-weighted images. Bone marrow and lymph node metastases were thus more clearly visible on the STIR images than on the T₂-weighted ones (Fig. 3-8).

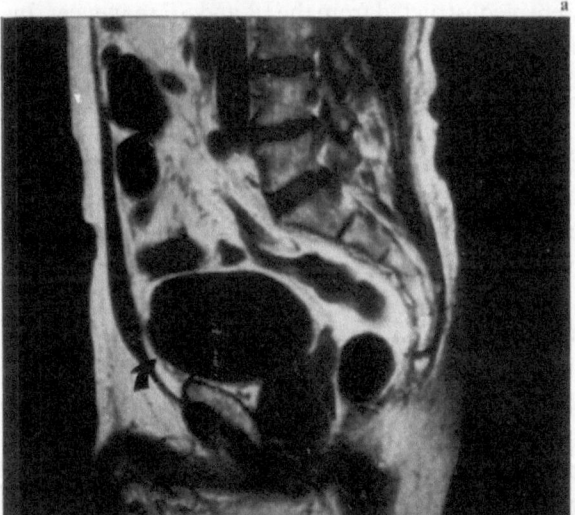
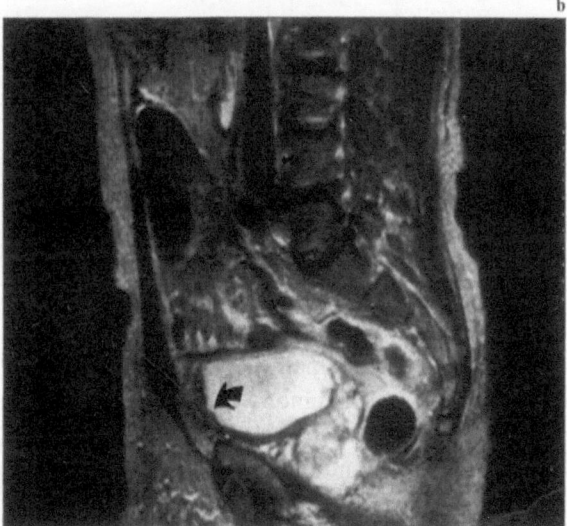

Fig. 3-7. (a) On the T1-weighted sagittal MR image (1.5 T; SE/650/30/2), a thickening of the ventral part of the bladder wall is visible (curved arrow). **(b)** On the T2-weighted image (SE/2000/100/2), this swelling has a raised signal intensity (arrow) in keeping with a tumor. The histologic diagnosis was, however, fibrosis with granulation and infected tissue (stage T0).

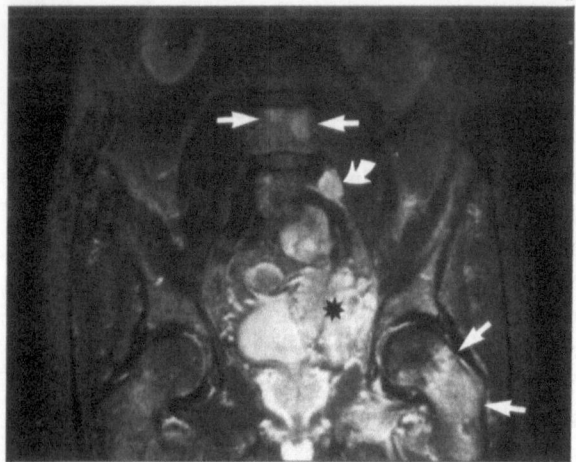 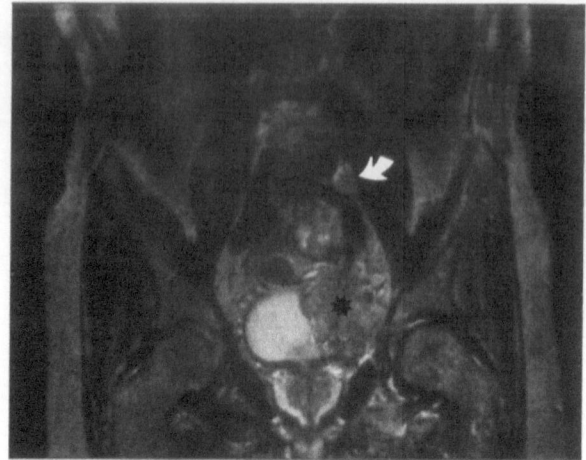

Fig. 3-8. (a) On the coronal MR image made by using the STIR sequence (1.5 T; IR/2000/100/30/2), primary tumor (*), lymph node metastases (curved arrow) and bone marrow metastases (straight arrows) can be clearly recognized from their high signal intensity. **(b)** On the SE image (1.5 T; SE/2000/100/2) the signal intensity of the tumor tissue is lower, and partly because of motion artifacts, the metastases in L4 cannot be seen. One also should be aware of the difference in signal strength of subcutaneous fat on the STIR and SE images.

Recently, it also became possible to reconstruct T_1, T_2 and proton-density images on the basis of a combination of two SE sequences. From these T_1-weighted, T_2-weighted and proton density images, images could be synthesized for every sequence desired. To demonstrate how the contrasts in the MR image varied and what the optimal sequences were, section 3.3.3.3 will describe the findings with this method in a patient with a large UBC with bone marrow metastases.

3.3.3.1 T_1 and T_2 calculations to optimize the pulse sequence

In 14 patients with UBC (10 men and 4 women), MR images were made to determine T_1 and T_2 values of tumor, fat, bladder wall and urine. The average age of the patients was 73 years. The final histologic diagnosis was transitional cell carcinoma (13 patients) and anaplastic carcinoma (1 patient). Tissue for histologic diagnosis was obtained by means of cystectomy (3 patients) or by deep transurethral resection (11 patients). At the time of the MR examination, the size (minimally 1.5 X 1.5 cm) and the exact location of the tumor were known.

A Philips 'superconductive' magnet with a field strength of 1.5 T was used (Gyroscan S15). From three series of T_1-weighted (SE/500/30/2) MR images, made in three planes perpendicular to each other, the slice giving the best view of the tumor was

determined. Then in 10 patients, an image of this slice was made with combined IR and SE sequences. The parameters for the IR and SE parts were IR/2220/380/30 and SE/680/30,60,90,120 respectively. The slice thickness was 10 mm; the matrix was 256 x 256.

In 4 other patients, instead of using the combined sequence, a T_2-weighted image was made with multiple echos (SE/2000/30,60,90,120,150,180,210,240). The imaging times for the mixed sequence and the T_2 sequence were each 15 min. 'T$_1$' and 'T$_2$' images were reconstructed from the IR and SE sequences. In these 'T$_1$' and 'T$_2$' images, each gray value represents a certain T_1 and a certain T_2 respectively.

Only T_2 images were reconstructed from the T_2-weighted SE sequences. The exact method of calculating these is beyond the scope of this book. The reader is, therefore, referred to the literature for further information.[113, 146]

The T_1 and T_2 values for perivesical fat, bladder wall, tumor and urine were measured on the T_1 and T_2 images. It was difficult to measure the very thin bladder wall (sometimes thinner than 5 mm). In order to obtain a reliable result, the T_1 and T_2 values were measured at three sites on the bladder wall in each patient. The average of these three measurements was taken as the final value. The T_1 and T_2 values times found are presented in Table 11, along

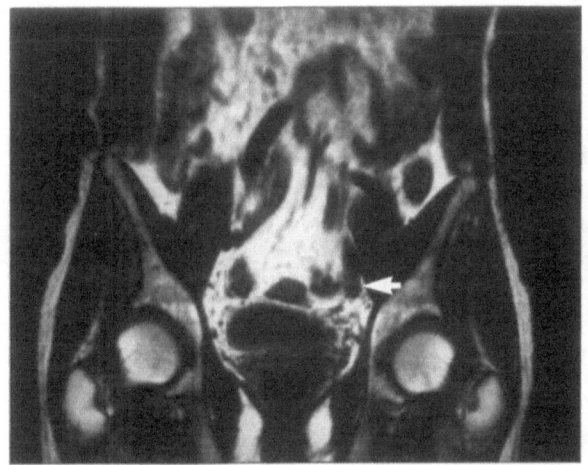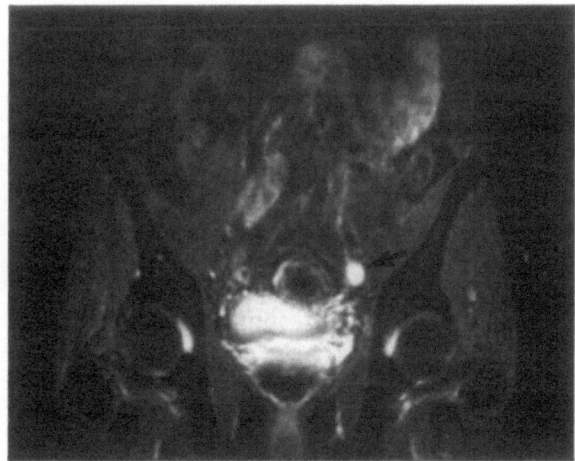

Fig. 3-9. (a) Owing to its poor signal, an enlarged node (arrow) is not very noticeable on the coronal MR image (1.5 T; SE/750/30/2).
(b) On the STIR image (1.5 T; IR/2000/120/30/2), this node has a very high signal intensity, in contrast to the very low signal intensity of fat.

with the standard deviations. Unfortunately, it was not possible to determine the exact proton density of the tissues in the pelvis.

Recently, by using a combination of two SE sequences (SE/750/30/2 and SE/2260/30,100/2), it became possible to reconstruct T_1, T_2, and proton-density images. The reader is referred to the literature for a description of the method.[8, 70, 145] This method was used to examine a patient, and the results were used for the reconstruction of 'contrast matrices' and for 'synthetic imaging' (see section 3.3.3.3).

3.3.3.2 *Pulse-sequence optimization by means of 'contrast matrices'*

In order to determine the optimal pulse sequence for differentiating two tissues, one must look at which sequence produces the maximal contrast between the two tissues. Also, one must consider whether the signal-to-noise ratio, which helps to determine the image quality, is sufficiently large.

On the basis of T_1, T_2, and proton-density values, matrices were reconstructed for various tissues in the pelvis (perivesical fat, tumor, bladder wall and urine), on which the difference in signal strength was visible for various sequence parameters. As the difference in signal strength is a measure of the final image contrast, these images are referred to as 'contrast

matrices' They show at which parameters (TR, TE, and/or TI) of a certain pulse sequence the contrast between two tissues is optimal. The reader is referred to the literature for descriptions of method[100] and formulas.[162] Because it was not possible to determine the exact proton-density of the tissues with the method earlier described, the proton-density was assumed to be the same for all. One can justify this assumption, as reported proton densities of the various tissues in the pelvis do not differ greatly.[75, 76] Furthermore, the proton density does not play a very large part in determining the optimal pulse sequence.[202]

Spin-echo sequence:

On the basis of the T_1 and T_2 values reported in Table 11, contrast matrices for tumor-fat, tumor-bladder wall and tumor- urine were constructed for the SE-pulse sequences (Fig. 3-10).

Here, the TR variation is indicated on the X-axis and the TE variation on the Y-axis. The black area in the contrast matrix indicates that there is no contrast. The white area represents high contrast. Sometimes several areas (Figs. 3-10d and 3-15d) have a contrast maximum or minimum. Some areas represent positive contrast, others negative contrast.

From these contrast matrices, one can deduce that the SE/500- 1100/<10 sequence is the optimal sequence for differentiating between *tumor and fat*. However, considering the limitations of the MRI equipment (TE smaller than 30 ms was not possible), in this study the *SE/750/30* sequence was chosen as the best.

To distinguish between *tumor and bladder wall*, the optimal sequence lies within the area: SE/>3600/100. For distinguishing between *tumor and urine* the best sequence is SE/>3800/>145. In order to use as few sequences as possible, an attempt was made to obtain the best contrast possible both between tumor and bladder wall and between tumor and urine with one sequence. Also, one had to take into account as short a TR as possible to limit the imaging time (see section 2.3.2). With this in mind, a TR of no longer than about 2000 ms was selected. From the contrast matrices, one can deduce that the *SE/2100/100* best fulfils the requirements. Furthermore, this sequence has an acceptable recording time: 15 min. With a TR greater than 2600 ms, the imaging time is about 20 min at least.

Inversion-recovery sequence:

The SE/750/30 sequence appears to be suitable for the recognition of bone marrow metastases and other abnormalities of bone marrow. On these images, however, bone marrow metastases, as well as other abnormalities (e.g., degenerative abnormalities, old traumata, local increases in density of bone) have a low signal intensity compared with the (fatty) bone marrow.

In order to be able to differentiate between bone marrow metastases and other abnormalities of the bone marrow, a sequence was sought in which tissues with a long T_1 and T_2 (tumor) have a very high signal intensity and surrounding structures (fat) a low signal intensity. For this purpose, a contrast matrix for tumor-fat was prepared for the (ST)IR-sequence

(Fig. 3-10d). The TR is kept constant (2000 ms). TI variation is indicated on the X-axis and TE variation on the Y-axis.

This contrast matrix contains three contrast optima: the right and left reflect where the fat signal intensity is higher than that of tumor. This contrast is comparable to the contrast of the T_1-weighted SE/750/30 sequence (tumor black, fat white). The median contrast optimum (100 < TI < 300) gives the desired difference in signal: tumor (long T_1 and T_2) has a very high signal intensity, while fat (short T_1 and T_2) gives hardly any signal.

One can deduce from the matrix that this contrast is obtained from the following sequences: *IR/2000/ 150-275/ ≤ 60*. It is precisely at these sequences that the signal of fat is optimally suppressed [TI = 0.59-0.69 times the T_1 value of fat (330 ms) = 194-270 ms (see section 2.3.2.2. and Table 11)]. One can also deduce that the TE selected should not be too long (≤ 60 ms).

3.3.3.3 *pulse-sequence optimization by means of 'synthetic imaging'*

From the T_1, T_2 and proton density images derived from two SE sequences (see section 3.3.3.1), MR images of a patient were compiled ('synthesized') with every desired pulse sequence and set of parameters. This method is called *'synthetic imaging.'* An explanation of this method is beyond the scope of this book. Those interested in further details are referred to the literature.[8] With synthetic imaging, one can gain some insight into how changes in pulse sequence or the adjustable parameters can alter the contrast on the MR image. An accompanying advantage of this method is that it can be applied simultaneously to various slices of the body. It also can be used to determine proton density.

Table 11 T_1 and T_2 tissue measurements.

	T_1 (9 patients)		T_2 (14 patients)	
perivesical fat	330	(52)	67	(2)
urinary bladder wall	1047	(48)	69	(2)
tumor	1153	(56)	107	(5)
urine	2343	(42)	340	(25)

( ) = standard deviation.

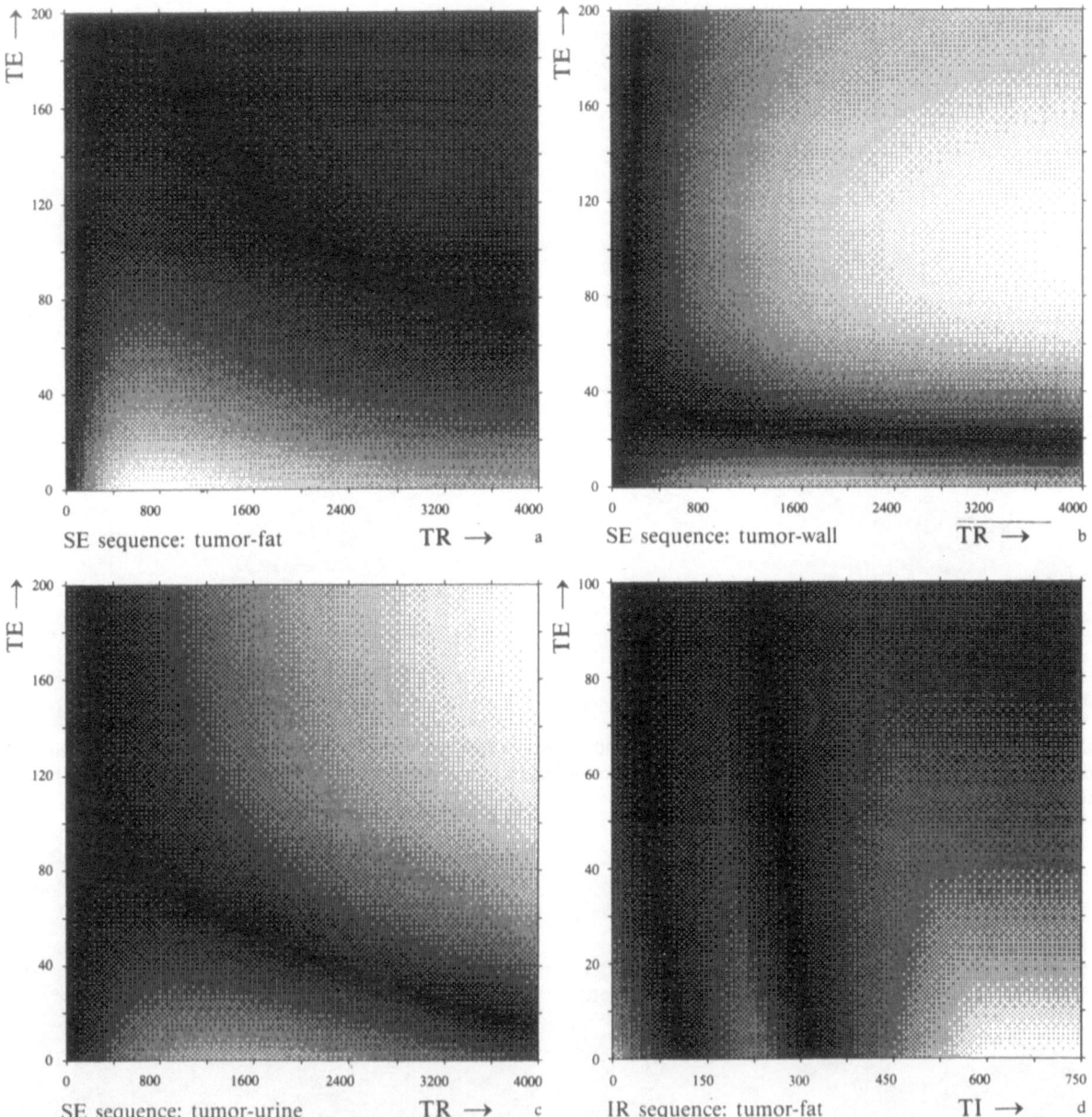

Fig. 3-10a-c. Contrast matrices for SE sequences. The TE variation (0-200 ms) is indicated on the Y-axis, the TR variation (0-4000 ms) on the X-axis. **(a)** Difference in signal between tumor and fat; **(b)** difference in signal between tumor and wall; **(c)** difference in signal between tumor and urine.

Fig. 3-10d. Contrast matrix for (ST)IR sequences (TR = 2000 ms) for difference in signal between tumor and fat. The TE variation (0-100 ms) is indicated on the Y-axis, the TI variation (0-750 ms) on the X-axis.

Fig. 3-11 shows the original MR images (SE/750/30/2 and SE/2260/100/2) made in patient v.M. who had a large UBC with bone marrow metastases. Fig. 3-12 shows the synthesized images with the same sequence parameters. That these images are more or less identical to the originals indicates that the calculation of the T_1, T_2 and proton-density images and the image synthesis are reliable.

Figs. 3-13 and 3-14 present series of synthesized ima-ges of *SE sequences* in which the TE and TR vary. The TR increases from left to right. The TE increases from bottom to top. Thus, the image at the bottom left is the most T_1-weighted and the image at the upperright is the most T_2-weighted.

In this patient, 'contrast matrices' were also made for SE sequences to measure the contrast between tumor and fat, tumor and bladder, wall and tumor and urine (Fig. 3-15a-c).

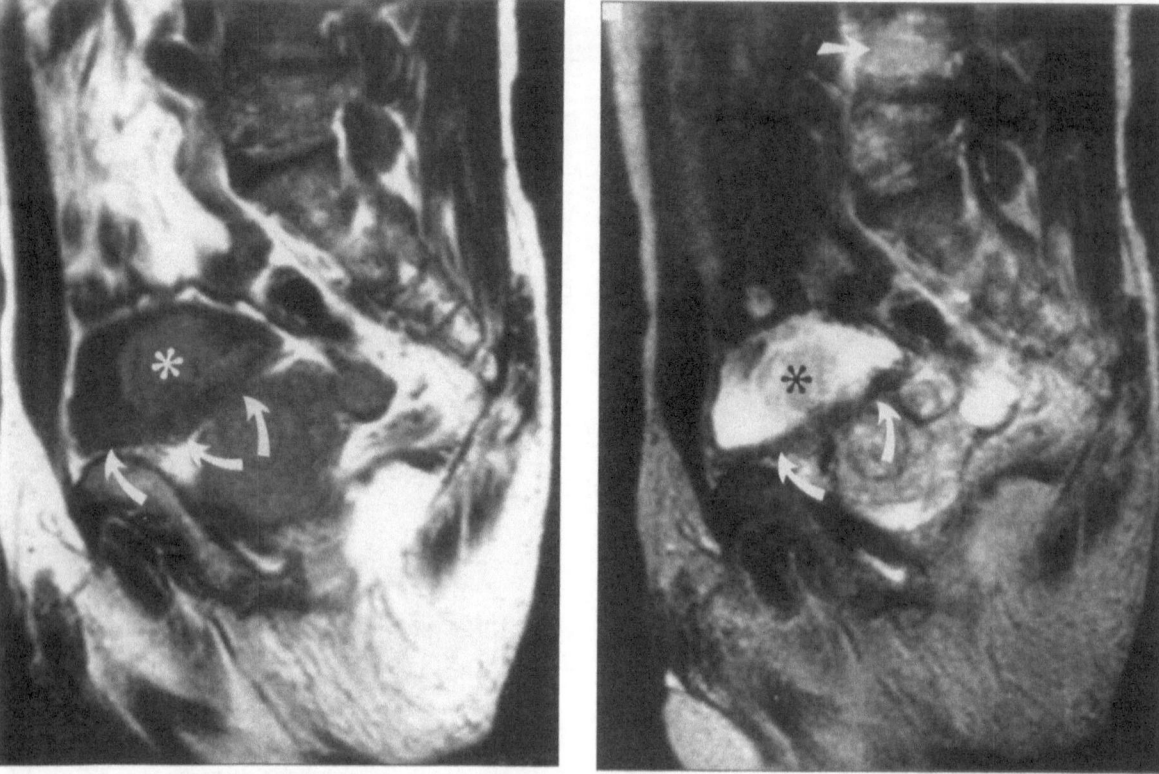

Fig. 3-11. 'Original' sagittal MR images: **(a)** (1.5 T; SE/750/30/2); **(b)** (1.5 T; SE/2260/100/2). A large papillar tumor is located in the center of the bladder (*). The wall is thickened at the floor of the bladder (curved arrows). Metastases can be found in the L4 body (straight arrows).

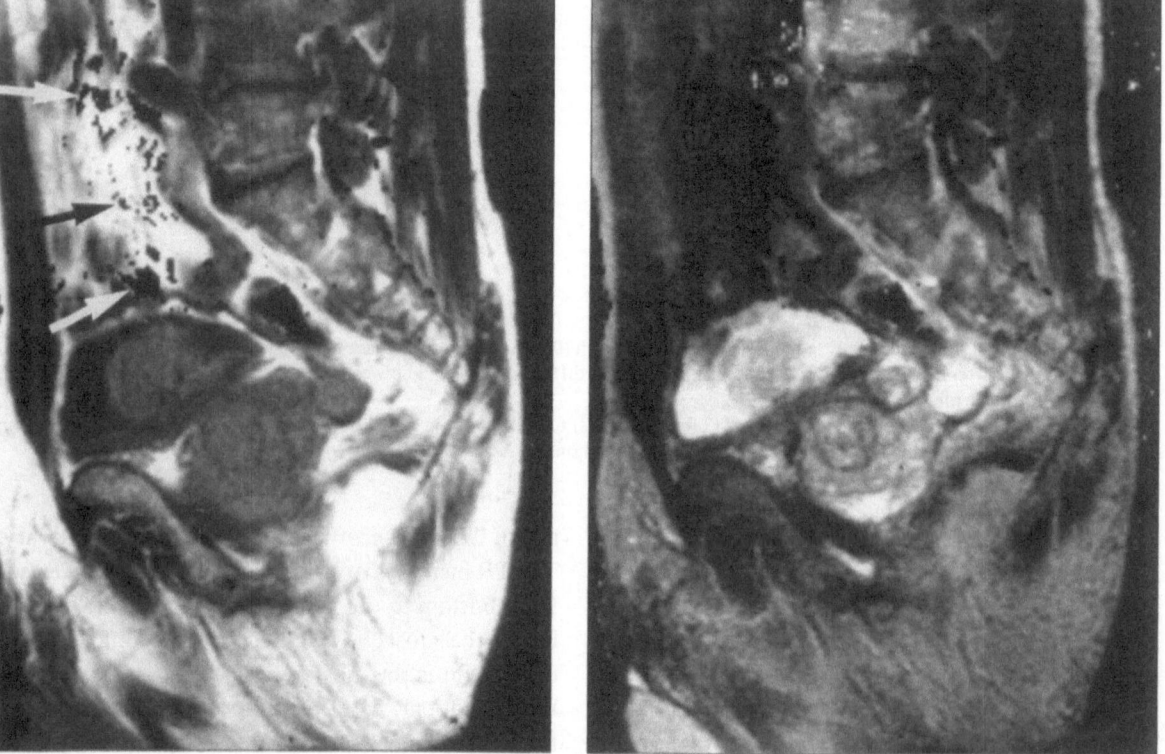

Fig. 3-12. Synthesized MR images. The sequences is identical to those in Fig. 3-11. The only difference are the calculation artifacts caused by motion (arrows).

In Figs. 3-13 and 3-14, one can see that the contrast between *tumor and fat* is optimal with the SE/1000/15 sequence and decreases as TE is extended. This is in accordance with what can be derived from the contrast matrix (Fig. 3-15a): this sequence lies in the white area.

The contrast between *tumor and bladder wall* first becomes visible on SE images with a TR $\geq$ 1000 ms and TE $\geq$ 60 ms. On images with a very long TE ($\geq$ 180 ms), the total signal decreases to such an extent that, in spite of the high contrast, the differentiation between wall and tumor becomes less. These findings are in accordance with those one can derive from the 'contrast matrix' (Fig. 3-15b): the optimal contrast is seen at a TR $\geq$ 1300 ms and a TE of 50-100 ms.

Finally, the difference between *urine and tumor* was assessed. From Figs. 3-13 and 3-14 it appears that at a very short TE ($<$15 ms) and a moderately long TR (1000 ms), the tumor clearly had a higher signal intensity than urine, a finding that agrees nicely with the white area at the bottom of the contrast matrix (Fig. 3-15c). Strong contrast occurred at a long TR ($\geq$ 2000 ms) and a long TE ($\geq$ 180 ms). This is in agreement with the white area on the right-hand side of the contrast matrix.

A contrast matrix (Fig. 3-15d) and synthesized images (Fig. 3-16) also were prepared for the *IR sequences*. The images were, however, of poorer quality because of motion artifacts. Figure 3-16 shows how the contrasts changed with variations in TI and TE. It is particularly obvious that fat gives hardly any signal at a TI of $\leq$ 250 ms. Conversely, the tumor produces a strong signal. This is in accordance with the median contrast optimum of the contrast matrix (Fig. 3-15d). At sequences with a TI of 250 ms and not too long a TE ($\leq$ 60 ms), tissues with a long T_1 and a long T_2 (E.G., tumor, vesicula seminalis, testicle, and urine) are highly apparent. With these parameters, a metastasis in vertebral body L4 became clearly visible. This metastasis was clearer on the IR/2000/250/60 sequence than on the T2-weighted SE sequence (SE/2000/90) so often used in other published studies [cf. Figs. 3-14 (*) and 3-15 (*)].

3.3.4 Interim conclusion

From this discussion, it follows that optimal imaging

of the urinary bladder and UBC requires a minimum of two sequences:

a. a *T_1-weighted sequence* to distinguish between fat and tumor (bladder wall) and between tumor and urine. The sequence described in the literature (SE/400-800/30) appears to satisfy these requirements and agrees with the sequence determined in section 3.3.3.2 (SE/750/15/2). Only the TE is somewhat shorter. Because of the limitation of the MR equipment, in the present study SE/750/30/2 had to be used. This sequence has a high signal-to-noise ratio and a short imaging time (5 min).

b. a *T_2-weighted sequence* to distinguish between bladder wall and tumor, tumor and urine, and tumor and fibrosis. The sequence described in the literature (SE/2000/100/2) seems to be quite suitable for this purpose and agrees with the sequence determined in section 3.3.3.2 (SE/2100/100). With SE/2000/150/2, it is essential to use a double surface coil (see section 3.4). Compared with the T_1-weighted sequence, the T_2-weighted sequence has a poorer signal-to-noise ratio and a longer imaging time (15 min).

Together with the T_2-weighted image, one can obtain a proton-weighted image (SE/2000/30/2) without extending the imaging time. This produces supplementary information about possible inflammation of the mucous membrane layer of the bladder wall.

If one suspects bone marrow and lymph node metastases, the *STIR sequence* (IR/2000/150-275/$\leq$60/2) has advantages over the T_2-weighted sequences. This sequence has a long imaging time (15 min) and a mediocre signal-to-noise ratio. These disadvantages are, however, more than compensated for by a reduction in motion and fat-shift artifacts.

3.4. Body-coil MRI versus (double) surface-coil MRI

The relaxation signals emitted are received by a coil and used to reconstruct an image. When creating an image of the body, a 'whole-body coil' is usually used. This is a cylindrical coil, about 45 cm in diameter, that completely surrounds the patient. As the distance between the signal source (patient) and the receiver coil diminishes, the signal-to-noise ratio and thus the quality of the image improves.[132] Coils that

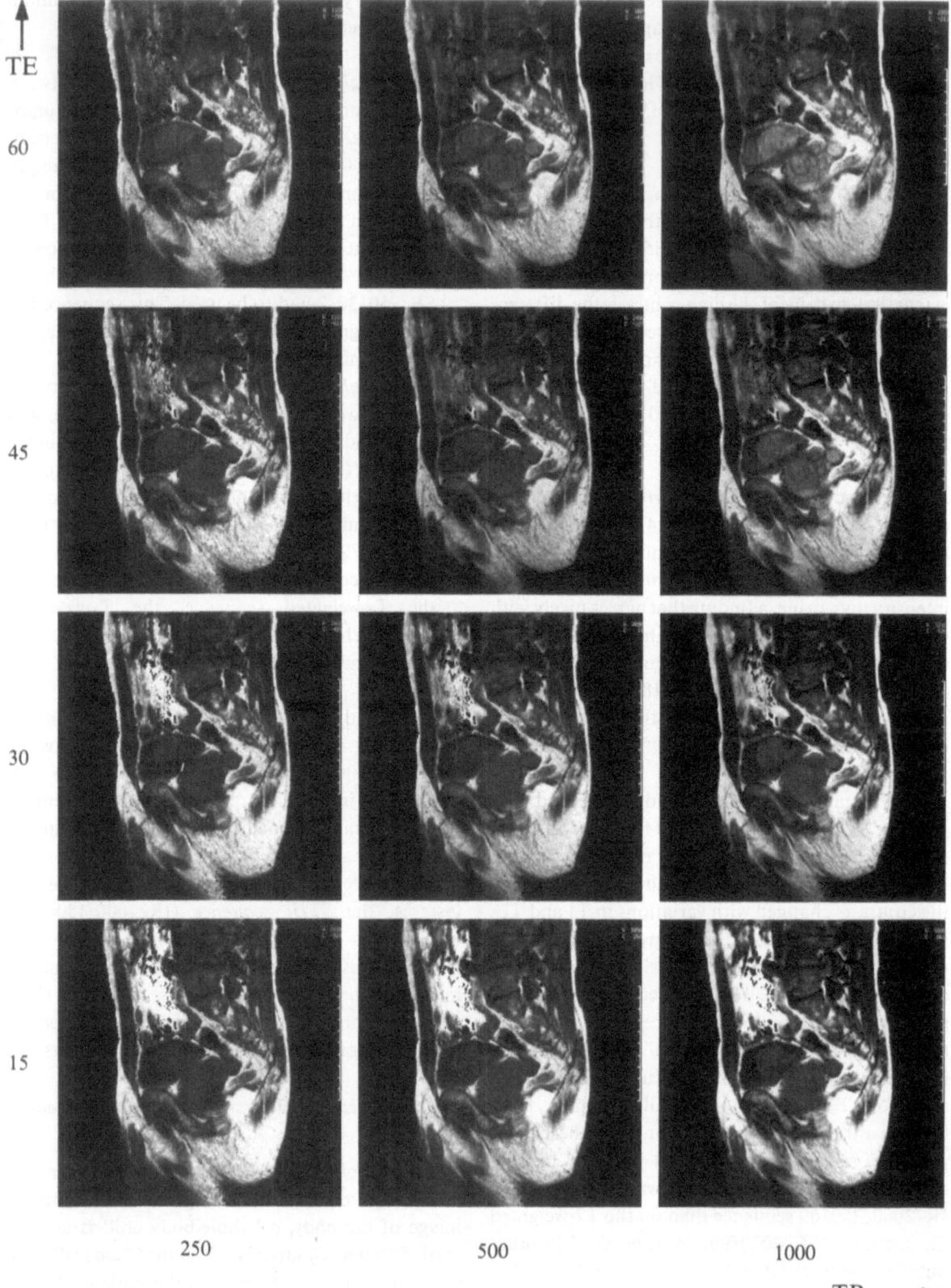

Fig. 3-13. Synthetic imaging for SE sequences. TE variation: 15-30-45-60 ms; TR variation 250-500-1000 ms.

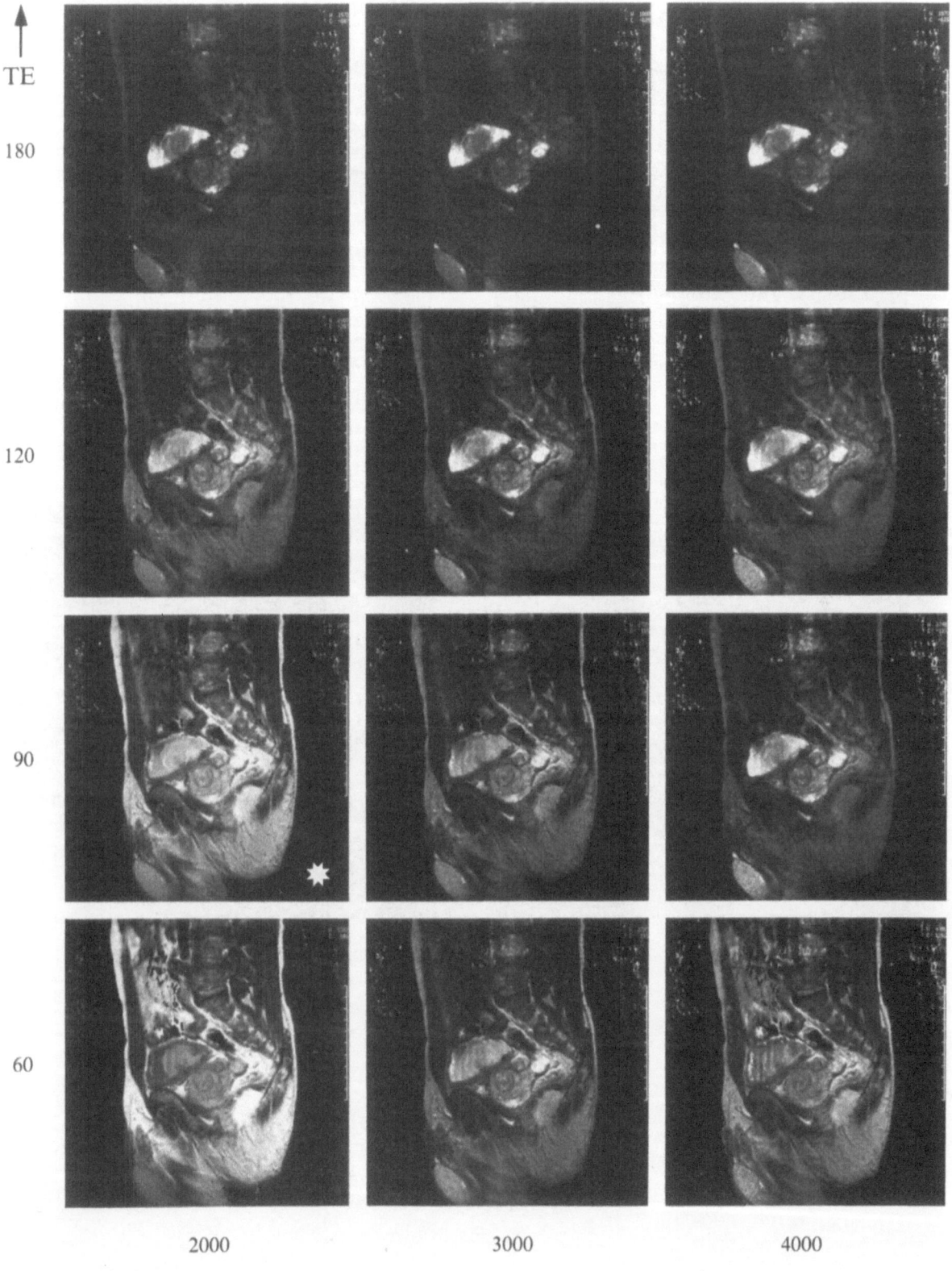

Fig. 3-14. Synthetic imaging for SE sequences. TE variation: 60-90-120-180 ms; TR variation: 2000-3000-4000 ms.

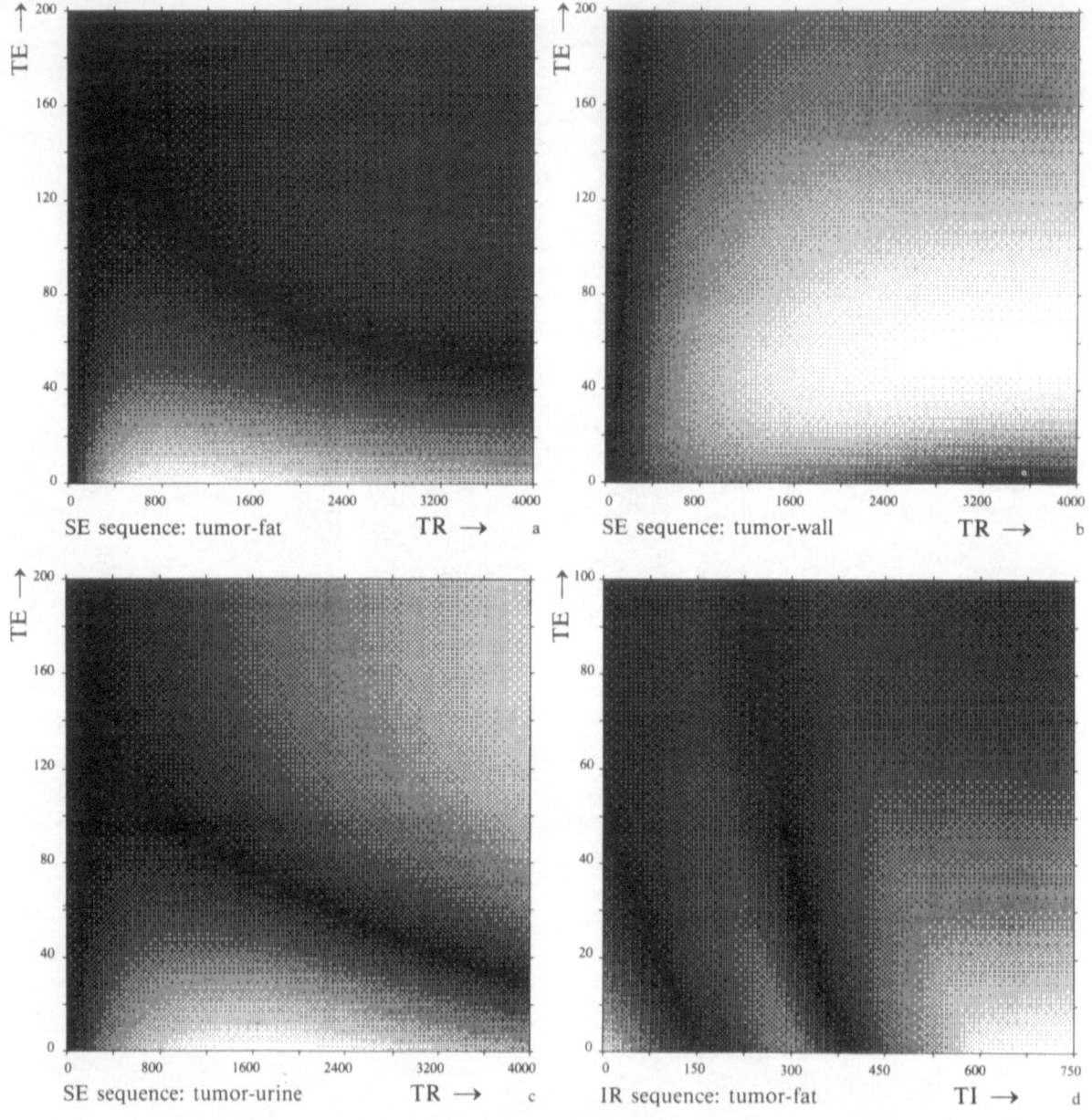

Fig. 3-15a-c. Contrast matrices for SE sequences of Figs. 3-13 and 3-14: **(a)** for difference in signal between tumor and fat, **(b)** tumor and wall, and **(c)** tumor and urine.
Fig. 3-15d. Contrast matrix for IR sequences for difference in signal between tumor and fat (TR = 2000 ms).

TI

500

250

100

50

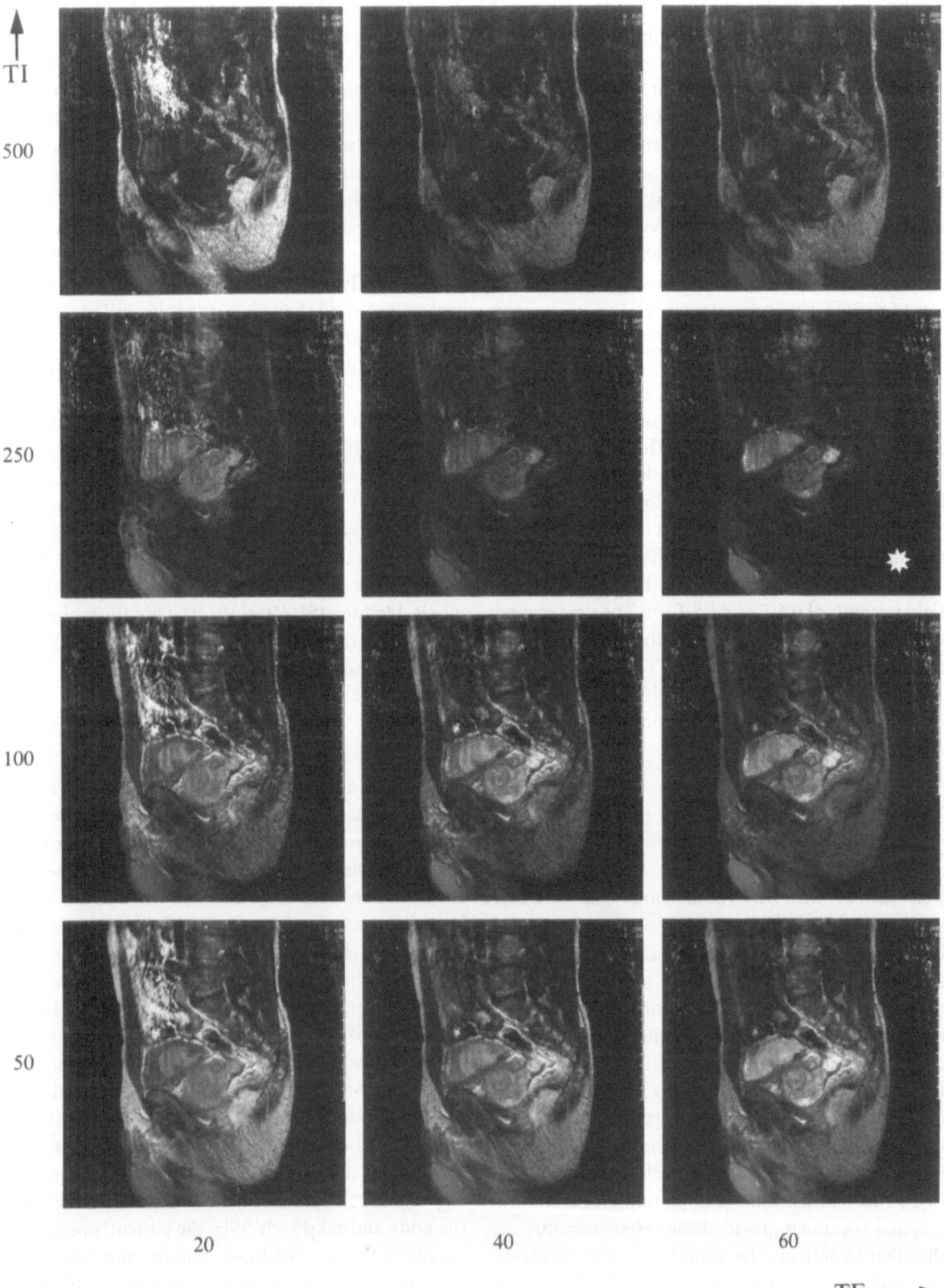

20   40   60

TE ⟶

Fig. 3-16. Synthetic imaging for IR sequences. TR = 2000 ms, TI variation: 50-100-250-500 ms; TE variation: 20-40-60 ms.

can be positioned close to the object to be imaged produce the best results. In practice, this is often on the patient's skin; hence the term 'surface coil.' Most surface coils consist of a single circular chain that is placed at a certain site on the patient's body. With these single coils, a clear improvement in signal-to-noise ratio and thus in image quality is achieved.[63, 66, 74, 147, 208, 227] However, these coils are not really suitable for creating images of pelvic structures, and particularly of the urinary bladder, because the signal-to-noise ratio reached is insufficient owing to loss of signal from deeper structures. In addition, the field of view is often too small.

To date, only one surface coil has been described with a double chain (Helmholtz coil).[199] When compared with images obtained with the whole-body coil, the images made with this double coil have a higher spatial resolution.[184, 186] However, because of the limited field of view, this coil is less suitable for staging UBC. In an effort to solve these problems, special double surface coils have been designed for field strength of 0.5 T and 1.5 T.[10,11] The next section will discuss the results of MRI with these double surface coils at field strengths of 0.5 T (24 patients) and 1.5 T (16 patients). The results with the double surface coil at 0.5 T have already been published[11] and are reported in section 3.4.1.

3.4.1   Results at a field strength of 0.5 T

3.4.1.1   *patients and methods*

In 24 patients with UBC (20 men and 4 women), MR images were made with the body coil and with a newly designed double surface coil. The average age of the patients was 61 years. The final histologic diagnosis was transitional cell carcinoma in 21 patients, anaplastic carcinoma in 2 patients, and squamous cell carcinoma in 1 patient. Tissue samples for histologic diagnosis were obtained by means of radical cystectomy (9 patients) or by transurethral deep tumor resection (15 patients). Pathologic staging was based on the TNM classification[215] (see Table 1 and Fig. 1). In 9 patients, the histopathologic data of the resected specimen provided the reference value. In the other 15 patients, the clinical staging method (see also section 1.2.2), backed up by the findings of at least 1.5 years follow-up, was the reference value. In 2 patients, transurethral resection was combined with a lymph node biopsy.

The MRI examination was performed with a Philips MR unit that contained a superconducting magnet (Gyroscan S5), operating at a field strength of 0.5 T. A 256 x 256 matrix was used. Use also was made of 'multiplanar' and 'multiecho' techniques. Buscopan® (butylscopamine) was administered to all patients according to the scheme described in section 3.2. Also, care was taken to ensure that the bladder was distended (see section 3.2). The MR staging was based on the scheme described by Fisher et al.[76] (see Table 12). A lymph node was considered to be abnormal/enlarged on the MR image if it was longer than 1.3 cm [57] and more than 1.0 cm in diameter.[43]

Body coil

By using the body coil, the bladder was located by obtaining a 10-mm-thick sagittal slice. Use was made of the following SE sequence: SE/250/30/1. This imaging took 1 min to obtain. Once the position of the bladder had been established, the slice thickness was reduced to 8 mm. Then a sequence with at least 8 images and a slice interval of 2 mm was made of the whole bladder (SE/500/30/2). This took about 5 min. In 2 patients, a T_2- weighted image (SE/2000/-30,100/2) also was acquired. This image took 17 min to obtain.

Surface coil

A special double surface coil was designed by Philips Medical Systems (Best).[10] This coil differs in size and shape from the Helmholtz coil. The latter consists of two circular coils of 17- cm diameter. The new surface coil (sandwich coil) consists of two rectangular coils measuring 20 x 40 cm (Fig. 3-17). One part is placed on the dorsal side and the other on the ventral side of the patient. The two parts are to a certain extent preformed to fit the contours of the body. Movement of the coil was prevented by tightening an adjustable belt. Excitation was achieved by emitting RF waves from the body coil. The sandwich coil only was used as a receiver.[26] The center of the coil was positioned 2 cm craniad to the symphysis pubis. In all patients, during the same examination, identical T_1-weighted images (SE/500/30/2) were made with the body and sandwich coils; the patient's position, the plane, the slice thickness, and the matrix were all the same. This was followed by making supplementary T_1- and T_2-weighted images in other planes with the sandwich coil. In 11 patients, the T_2-weighted sequence was SE/2000/30,100/2, in 6 it

Table 12   **MR staging system according to Fischer[76] (T stages).**

T stages:	Findings on MRI
Tis	Too small to be visualized.
T1	Tumor limited to bladder wall; exterior of bladder wall is normal. This normal bladder wall has a low signal intensity on T_2 weighted images.
T2	Same as T1.
T3A	Considerable tumor invasion of the bladder wall, seen as area of high signal intensity spreading throughout the entire bladder wall, but not as far as the perivesical fat. The remaining, unaffected part of the bladder wall can still be recognized by its lower signal intensity.
T3B	Interruption of the normal bladder wall (visible in at least two planes) and abnormal tissue outside the bladder wall in the perivesical fat.
T4A	Abnormal signal intensity, spreading to nearby organs (e.g., seminal vesicles, prostate, and rectum).
T4B	Abnormal signal intensity, spreading to pelvic cavity or abdominal wall.

was SE/2000/30,60/2, and in 7 it was SE/2000/30, 150/2. Because the examination took too long (17 min), an identical T_2-weighted image with the body coil only was made in 2 patients.

Comparison of body coil and surface coil

In order to quantify the improvement in signal-to-noise ratio, the signal intensity and the standard deviation (noise) of certain areas was measured.

The ability to distinguish a bladder tumor on T_1-weighted images is determined by the difference between the signal intensity of the tumor and that of the surrounding tissues (i.e. bladder content, bladder wall, and perivesical fat). Because it is very difficult to describe a sufficiently large region of interest in the thin bladder wall and bladder tumor to allow

accurate measurement of signal intensity, the signal intensity of the urine (Iu) and that of the perivesical fat (Iv) was determined. The average of these two measurements was used as an indication of the signal intensity of the tumor region. The signal intensity of an area outside the patient (background) (Ia) was subtracted from this. To determine noise, the standard deviation of the urine in the bladder was measured (SDu). Although one patient had severe hematuria, this did not appear to affect the homogeneity of the bladder content. As urine is normally a homogeneous mass, the standard deviation of urine was regarded as a reliable indicator of noise in this area.

The SDu provides a more accurate measure of noise than does the often used standard deviation of background.[184] The signal-to-noise ratio was determined according to the following formula for both body-coil and sandwich-coil images:

$$\text{SNratio} = \frac{\frac{1}{2}(\text{Iv} + \text{Iu}) \text{ minus Ia}}{\text{SDu}}$$

Identical regions of interest were used for both the body coil and the sandwich coil.

The identical T_1-weighted images, made with the body coil and sandwich coil, and the other MR images (made with the sandwich coil only), were evaluated retrospectively by three radiologists who had no prior knowledge of the final staging results. If there was a difference in interpretation of the MR images, the final staging was established after discussion.

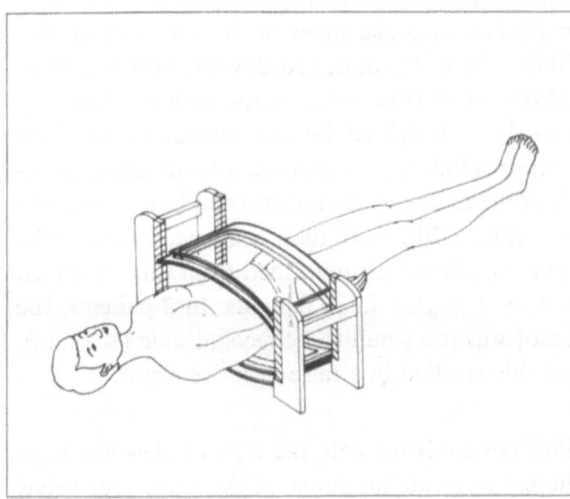

Fig. 3-17. Diagram of the 0.5 T-sandwich coil.

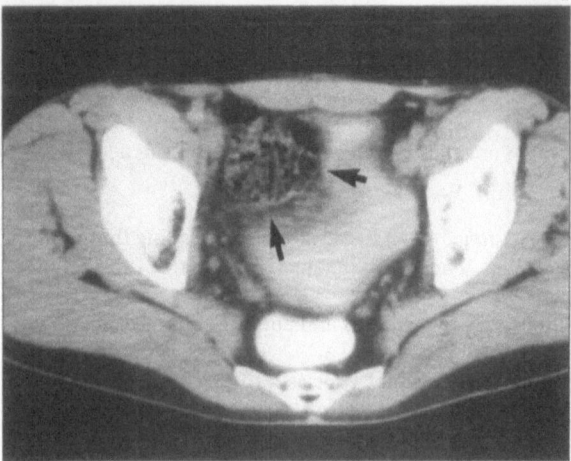 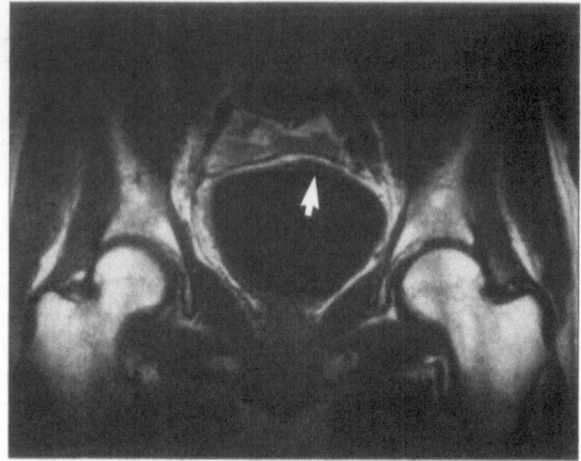

Fig. 3-18. (a) CT scan taken through the dome of the bladder reveals an impression due to a bowel loop (arrows), but no tumor. **(b)** MR image (0.5 T; SE/500/30/2) in the coronal plane reveals a flat tumor (arrow). This was verified histologically (stage T1).

3.4.1.2 *results*

The improvement in signal-to-noise ratio with the sandwich coil varied from 4.3 to 1.2 (average 1.9). This was a definite improvement over the visualization of anatomic structures with body-coil MRI. In Table 13, the staging results with the identical T_1-weighted MR images obtained with body coil and sandwich coil are presented and compared with the histopathologic findings of cystectomy or the clinical staging method (including follow-up). Five (21%) of the 24 patients were understaged with the sandwich coil MRI; overstaging did not occur. With the body coil, understaging was found in 10 patients (42%) and overstaging in 1 (4%). Thus, staging based on sandwich-coil MRI is significantly better ($P \leq .10$, chi-square test) than staging based on body-coil MRI.

In two patients, small tumors (<7-mm diameter) were detected with either the sandwich coil or the body coil. In another two patients, two small tumors (7 and 12 mm in diameter) were missed with the body coil, but detected with the sandwich coil. The high spatial resolution achieved with the sandwich coil is illustrated by the ability to distinguish a very small, thin lesion (Fig. 3-18).

The body coil understaged an abnormality (stage T3B) in one patient, while sandwich-coil MRI staged it correctly (stage T4B). In one patient, tumor infiltration into the wall of the rectum was not discovered with the body coil, whereas sandwich-coil MR images displayed this lesion clearly (Fig. 3-19). This extra

finding did not, however, affect the final staging of the tumor.

In the 2 patients in whom identical T_2-weighted sequences were used (patients 8 and 11), the image quality obtained with the sandwich coil was much better. In patient 8, a tumor staged as T2 could differentiated correctly from stage T3A with the sandwich coil, something that was not possible with the body coil.

Lymph node metastases were found in seven patients. In four of these, the lymph nodes also were enlarged. In two of these patients, the enlarged lymph nodes were visible on the sandwich-coil images, but not on the body-coil images. The other three patients had metastases in normal-sized lymph nodes. The improvement in signal-to-noise ratio enabled one to make images with a very long TE and TR (SE/2000/30,100 or 150/2) with a very good spatial resolution (Fig. 3-4). On the basis of these very strongly T_2-weighted images, thanks to the high spatial resolution, it was possible to determine accurately the extent of tumor invasion into the muscle layer (Fig. 3-20). With these sequences, stage Ta-T2 tumors could be distinguished from tumors staged as T3A or higher in 11 patients. In 2 patients, the tumor was too small to be recognizable (<7 mm), and this resulted in a false-negative result.

With the sandwich coil, the field of view was large enough to create an image of the entire true pelvis with a minimum of sequences (Fig. 2-13). The blad der and lymph nodes in the true pelvis and along the iliac vessels could be displayed with one sequence. A minimum of 18 slices in the transverse plane (8-mm thick, 2-mm intervals) could be made with one sequence. The sandwich coil had an RF-field sensitivity that was homogeneous in the entire area imaged in the transverse plane (Fig. 3-21b). Conversely, images made with a single, circular surface coil, like the one described by Fisher et al. [74], demonstrated a strong deterioration in signal on the dorsal side, which resulted in poor delineation of the tumor (Fig. 3-21a). Furthermore, the field of view with this single circular coil was limited, and so it was impossible to evaluate bladder and iliac lymph nodes on the same image.

3.4.1.3 *discussion*

As a result of therapeutic policy, only a few patients underwent cystectomy (nine patients). Of these, one had a tumor staged as T2, two patients had a stage T3A tumor, three a stage T3B, and three a stage T4B.

With identical T_1-weighted images, the higher spatial resolution obtained with the sandwich coil resulted in better discrimination of the tumor from the perivesical fat and the bladder lumen. This indicates that tumor staging with the double surface coil is more reliable (79% correctly staged) than with the body coil (54% correctly staged). The staging results for the double surface coil are better than those reported for the body coil: 64% [6] and 70%.[188] Had these authors included patients with small lesions [6] or with microscopic lymph node metastases [6, 188] in their series, the percentages found would have been even lower. Fisher et al. [76] achieved a very high accuracy (86%) when they used body-coil MRI to stage UBC. This study, however, only included patients with tumors staged as T3A or higher.

Table 13 Results of staging with T_1-weighted body coil and sandwich coil MR images (0.5 T).

Patient no.	body coil	sandwich coil	pathologic stage
	TNM stage		
1	T3B	T4B	T4B
2	T4B	T4B	T4B
3	T3B	T3B	T3B
4	T3B,N2	T3B,N2	T3B,N2
5	T3B	T3B	T3B,N2
6	≤T3A	≤T3A	T3A,N1
7	≤T3A	≤T3A	T3A,N2
8	≤T3A	≤T3A	T2
9	T4B	T4B,N2	T4B,N2
10	T3B	T3B,N2	T3,N2
11	T3B	T3B	T3
12	T4A,N3	T4A,N3	T4A,N3
13	≤T3A	≤T3A	T1
14	normal	≤T3A	T2
15	≤T3A	≤T3A	T1
16	normal	normal	T1
17	≤T3A	≤T3A	T1
18	≤T3A	≤T3A	T1
19	≤T3A	≤T3A	T1
20	normal	≤T3A	T1
21	normal	normal	T1
22	≤T3A	≤T3A	T1
23	≤T3A	≤T3A	T1
24	≤T3A	≤T3A	T1

Remarks: The TNM staging system was used. All patients had tumors staged as N0, M0 unless otherwise stated. N+ = lymph node metastasis proved by percutaneous biopsy. In patients 1-9, radical cystectomy was the reference; in patients 10-24, the clinical staging method (incl. follow-up > 1.5 years) served as reference.

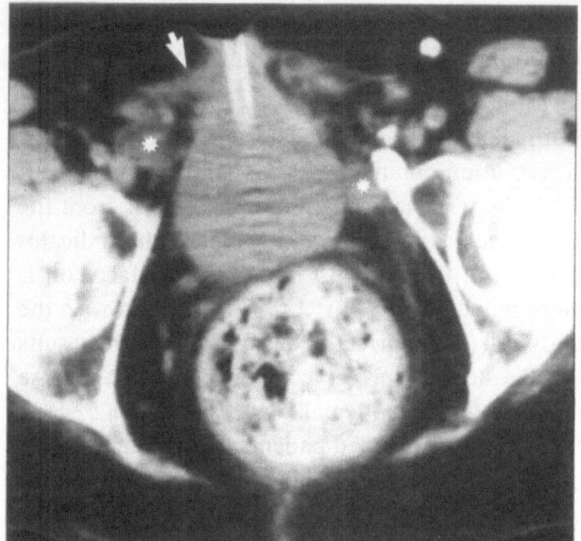

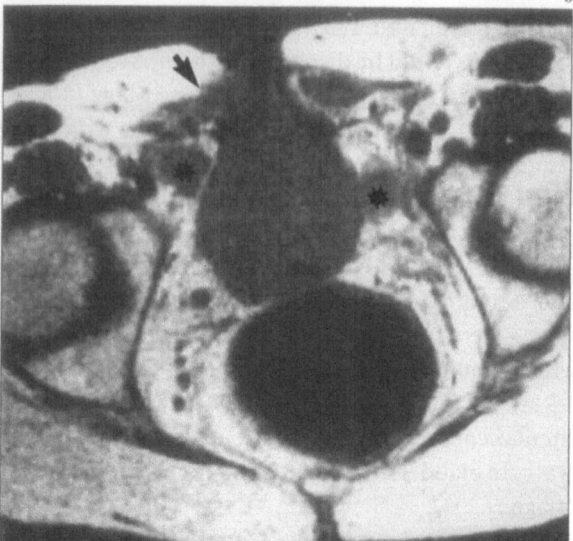

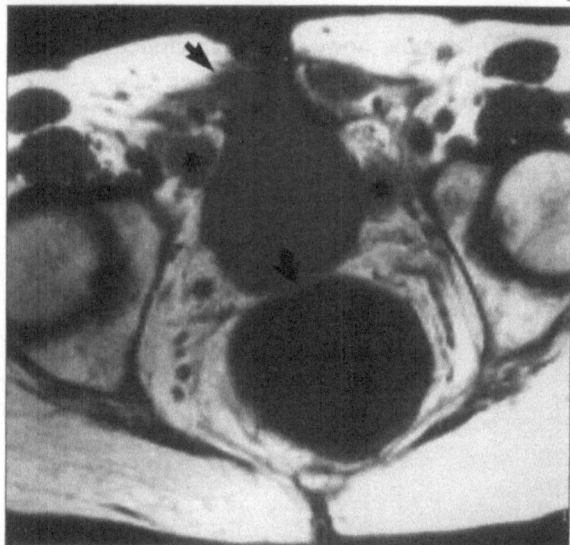

Fig. 3-19. Patient with squamous cell carcinoma of the bladder with a suprapubic catheter. The bladder lumen cannot be distinguished **(a)** on the CT scan or **(b)** on the MR images made with the body coil and **(c)** the double surface coil (0.5 T; SE/500/30/2). There is tumor infiltration around the suprapubic catheter (arrow) and perivesically (*). On **(a)** and **(b)**, there is no interruption of the fat layer between bladder with tumor and rectum wall. This argues against invasion of the rectum wall. **(c)** On the MR image made with the double surface coil, interruption of this fat layer *can* be seen (curved arrow), which is indicative of invasion of the rectum wall. This was confirmed at autopsy.

In order to determine the depth of invasion into the bladder wall, one must use a very long TE at a field strength of 0.5 T (150 ms, see section 3.3). As smaller relaxation signals are received at a longer TE, the signal and accordingly the signal- to-noise ratio decrease. The latter results in poor image quality. For this reason, very long TEs (e.g. ≥150 ms) have not been used. The improvement in signal-to-noise ratio and thus in spatial resolution that can be achieved with the sandwich coil allows one to obtain an image with a good spatial resolution even at a TE of 150 ms. The results of sandwich coil MR with long TEs (SE/2000/150/2) show that it is feasible to obtain a reliable determination of the depth of tumor invasion into the muscle layer.

3.4.2 Results at a field strength of 1.5 T

As described in the preceding section (3.4.1), separate double surface coils have to be made for use at 0.5 T and 1.5 T. A study like the one described earlier has been performed at a field strength of 1.5 T in 16 patients. Next, we will discuss briefly the differences with 0.5 T.

3.4.2.1 *patients and methods*

In 16 patients with carcinoma of the urinary bladder (13 men and 3 women), MR images were made with both the body coil and the double 1.5-T surface coil. The average age of the patients was 64 years. The histologic diagnosis was transitional cell carcinoma

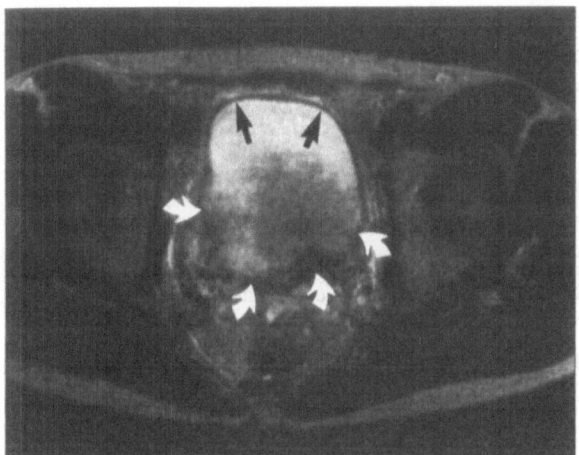

Fig. 3-20. MR image in the transverse plane with a very long TE and using the double surface coil (0.5 T; SE/2000/150/2). The normal bladder wall (straight arrows) is visible as a thin layer with low signal. This is interrupted on the dorsal side by tumor (curved arrows) (stage T3A). See also Fig. 6-1.

The examination was performed with a Philips MR system with a superconducting magnet at a field strength of 1.5 T (Gyroscan S15). The imaging technique was the same as that used at 0.5 T (see section 3.4.1.1). In all patients, two identical T_1-weighted images were made with both the body coil and the surface coil. Then two T_1-weighted and one T_2-weighted images were made in two other planes by using the double surface coil only. In 14 patients, the imaging parameters of the T_2-weighted series were in accordance with the description in section 3.4.1.1 (SE/2000/30,100/2). In 2 patients, an SE/3000/30, 100/1 sequence was used (see section 3.3.2).

in all cases. In 4 patients, it appeared that at the time of examination there was no longer any residual tumor tissue. This was the result of a total transurethral tumor resection or of the effect of radiotherapy or chemotherapy (see also Chapter 5).

Radical cystectomy was performed in 4 patients. The histopathologic findings on the resected specimen served as the reference value in these patients. The reference for the other patients was the clinical staging method backed up by follow-up lasting 6 months to 2.5 years.

The double surface coil for 1.5 T was not manufactured under optimal circumstances as was the case for 0.5 T (Philips Medical Systems, Best), but was constructed at the MRI Institute of the University Hospital, Utrecht. The choice of electronic components was limited and therefore suboptimal. Neither were tuning and matching as easy as with the 0.5 T sandwich coil. As the lymph nodes and the aorta bifurcation had to be displayed by using the 1.5-T coil, the measurements of this coil were different from those of the 0.5-T sandwich coil: the 1.5-T double surface coil consists of a combination of two rectangular coils measuring 30 x 40 cm (instead of 20 x 40 cm). Moreover, the 1.5-T coil was made of a more flexible material than the 0.5-T coil.

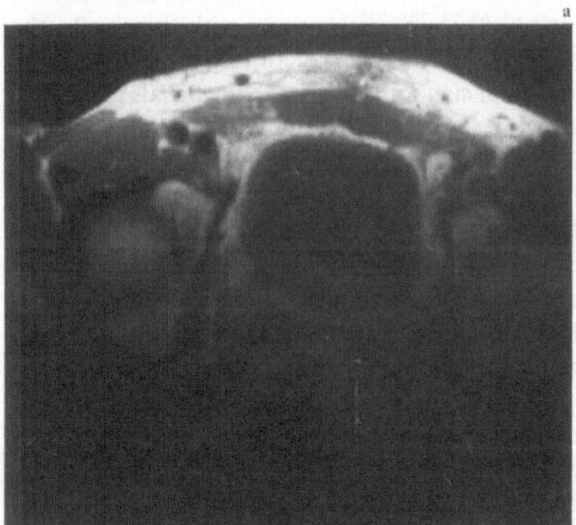

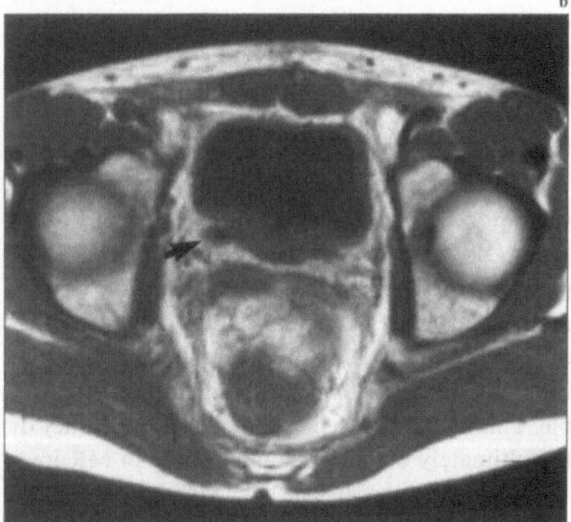

Fig. 3-21. (a) MR image in the transverse plane, made with a single circular surface coil (0.5 T; SE/500/30/2). This shows a loss of signal intensity on the dorsal side, and the field of view is limited. Neither the tumor on the dorsal side nor the dilated right ureter are visible. (b) MR image made with a double surface coil (same parameters) shows a homogeneous RF field and an adequate field of view. The tumor and dilated ureter (arrow) can be recognized.

The pathologic staging, the interpretation of the MR images, and the analysis of the images were identical to the procedures at 0.5 T.

3.4.2.2 *results*

The improvement in signal-to-noise ratio when the double surface coil was used rather than the body coil varied from 2.7 to 0.7 (an average of 1.25). This resulted in a better image quality in seven patients. Table 14 presents the staging results of the identical T_1-weighted MR images obtained with body coil and double surface coil. In 1 of the 16 patients, overstaging occurred with the double surface coil. Understaging was not encountered. With the body coil, overstaging was found in 2 and understaging in 1 patient. The series is too small to allow any conclusion about a significant improvement in staging accuracy as a result of using the double surface coil.

In 6 patients, lymph node metastases were found. This diagnosis was established in 1 patient during cystectomy, in 1 patient after percutaneous biopsy, and in the others on the basis of lymphographic examination, combined with follow-up. In all 6 patients, the pathologically enlarged nodes were found on the MR images made with the surface coil. In 1 patient, these nodes were not recognizable on images made with the body coil. The area imaged with the 1.5-T double surface coil was larger than that with the 0.5-T sandwich coil. Structures lying beside the distal aorta and vena cava inferior, such as lymph nodes, were also displayed in this way (see Fig.4-4).

3.4.2.3 *discussion*

Unfortunately, the number of patients in this group who underwent cystectomy is even smaller than it was in the group described in section 3.4.1. This group also included a relatively large number of patients with deep tumor infiltration and lymph node metastases (see Table 14). The reference value of the group, who did not undergo cystectomy and in whom the follow-up period was short, is less reliable. This will influence in particular the accuracy of the ultimately obtained stagings (94% in MR images, made with the surface coil; 81% in MR images made with the body coil).

Nevertheless, the results of this part of the study give a good indication of the improvement in MRI when

the double surface coil is used at 1.5 T: in seven patients the quality of the image was definitely better, and this resulted in more accurate tumor staging in two patients.

The staging results obtained for the group of patients with the surface coil at 1.5 T are better than those obtained with the sandwich coil at 0.5 T (accuracy 94% and 79% respectively). The effect of the higher field strength is probably of relevant here. In section 3.5, we will come back to the differences in tumor staging between patients investigated at field strength of 0.5 T and 1.5 T.

The improvement in signal-to-noise ratio of the sandwich coil (0.5 T) is clearly greater than that of the double surface coil (1.5 T) (2.0 and 1.25, respectively). There are a number of reasons for this:
1. the tuning and matching is much more critical at higher field strengths, and this was not always optimal with the 1.5-T coil;
2. the choice of electronic components was not optimal; there must have been definite consequences for the signal-to-noise ratio, and
3. the field of view of the 1.5-T coil was larger.

3.4.3   Interim conclusion

The quality of MR images of abdominal structures can definitely be improved by using single circular surface coils. This is due to a better signal-to-noise ratio.[63, 66, 74, 208, 227] However, with these coils, the sensitivity for deeper structures decreases, resulting in a lower signal-to-noise ratio for signals from these structures. Accordingly, this type of coil is not suitable for producing good images of the urinary bladder (Fig. 3-21a). So far, one double surface coil has been described: the Helmholtz coil.[184,186] The field of view of this coil is, however, also limited, making it less suitable for staging UBC. The new double surface coils have a larger field of view, enabling one to generate an image of the entire true pelvis and the lower part of the abdomen in one sequence. Images made with the new double surface coils also have a definitely higher signal-to-noise ratio than do the body-coil MR images. This is particularly true for the images made with the sandwich coil (0.5 T).

If the acquisition time is kept the same, the higher signal- to-noise ratio produces images with better spatial resolution. This leads to more accurate staging of UBC. In particular, the depth of invasion of the tumor into the bladder wall can be determined more accurately with this coil. The double surface coil used here at a field strength of 1.5 T did not produce much improvement in image quality because of its poor quality.

The next section will deal whether the staging results obtained without use of a double surface coil at 1.5 T are better than those obtained at 0.5 T *with* the use of a double surface coil.

3.5 Comparison of staging results at 0.5 T versus 1.5 T

3.5.1 Introduction

In order to obtain an insight into the differences between MRI of UBC at field strengths of 0.5 and 1.5 T, the staging results at these field strengths are compared. For a review of the total patient group, the reader is referred to section 5.1.

In 33 patients, an adequate MR examination was performed at a field strength of 0.5 T, and in 101

others at a field strength of 1.5 T. In all patients investigated at 0.5 T, the sandwich coil was used (see section 3.4.1). In the 1.5-T MR examinations, incidental use was made of a suboptimal double surface coil (see section 3.4.2).

3.5.2 Patients, methods and results

Patients and methods are described in Chapter 5. The results are presented in Tables 15A and 15B. Because it is not possible to distinguish between tumor stages Ta, T1 and T2 with MRI,[76] these are grouped together as stage Ta-T2.

The histopathologic findings of cystectomy/autopsy or those of the clinical staging method, backed up by follow-up, were used as reference values (see section 5.1). These patients, who underwent cystectomy or obduction, are represented by asterics. The patients with tumors in stages T2 or higher, who did not undergo cystectomy or autopsy, are indicated in Tables 15A and 15B in italics. The reference value for the latter group of patients is unreliable (see Chapter 5).

Table 14   Results of staging of T_1-weighted body coil and sandwich coil MR images (1.5 T).

Patient no.	TNM stage		
	body coil	sandwich coil	pathologic stage
1	T3B	T4B,N4	T3B,N4
2	T4B,M+	T4B,M+	T4B,M+
3	≤T3A	≤T3A	T3A
4	T3B	T3B	T3B
5	fibrosis	fibrosis	T0
6	normal	normal	T0
7	mucosal edema,N4	mucosal edema,N4	T0,N4
8	T3B	T3B	T0
9	≤T3A	≤T3A	T1
10	≤T3A	≤T3A	T1
11	≤T3A	≤T3A	T2-3A
12	≤T3a	≤T3A	T3
13	≤T3A,N4,M+	≤T3A,N4,M+	T3,N4,M+
14	T4A,N4	T3B,N4	T3,N+
15	T3B,N4	T3B,N4	T3,N4
16	T4A,N4	T4A,N4	T4A,N4

Remarks: The TNM staging system was used. All patients had tumors staged as N0, M0 unless otherwise stated. N+ = lymph node metastasis proved by percutaneous biopsy. In patients 1-4, radical cystectomy was the reference; in patients 5-16, the clinicl staging method (incl. follow-up from 9 monds - 3 year) served as reference.

Table 15 A   Results of staging with MRI at 0.5 T (T stages).

MRI stage	cystectomy / clinical staging method							
	T0	Ta-1	T2	T3A	T3B	T4A	T4B	
T0	5	2	—	—	—	—	—	
Ta-2	2* + 1	10	1*	—	—	—	—	
T3A	—	—	—	*2* + 3*	—	—	—	
T3B	—	—	—	—	2*	—	—	
T4A	—	—	—	—	—	1* + 2	—	
T4B	—	—	—	—	—	—	2*	
	8	12	1	5	2	3	2	33

* = cystectomy was the reference (10 patients); the reference for the other patients was the clinical staging method (incl. follow-up).

italics = reference unreliable.

Table 15 B   Results of staging with MRI at 1.5 T (T stages).

MRI stage	cystectomy / clinical staging method							
	T0	Ta-1	T2	T3A	T3B	T4A	T4B	
T0	3* + 13	1	—	—	—	—	—	
Ta-2	3* + 2	3* + 21	1* + 1	*1*	—	—	—	
T3A	1	*1*	2	3* + 9	—	—	—	
T3B	2 + 2	—	—	3* + 8	8* + 1	—	—	
T4A	—	—	—	2	1*	4 + 1*	—	
T4B	—	—	—	—	—	—	*4* + 2*	
	26	26	4	24	10	5	6	101

* = cystectomy was the reference (30 patients); the reference for the other patients was the clinical staging method (incl. follow-up).

italics = reference unreliable.

Table 16 A   Results of staging with MRI at 0.5 T (N stages).

MRI stage	cystectomy / autopsy staging or lymphography (incl. follow-up)		
	N0	N+	number of patients
N0	6	3	9
N+	0	6	6
n	6	9	15

Table 16 B   Results of staging with MRI at 1.5 T (N stages).

MRI stage	cystectomy / autopsy staging or lymphography (incl. follow-up)		
	N0	N+	number of patients
N0	34	0	34
N+	0	9	9
n	34	9	43

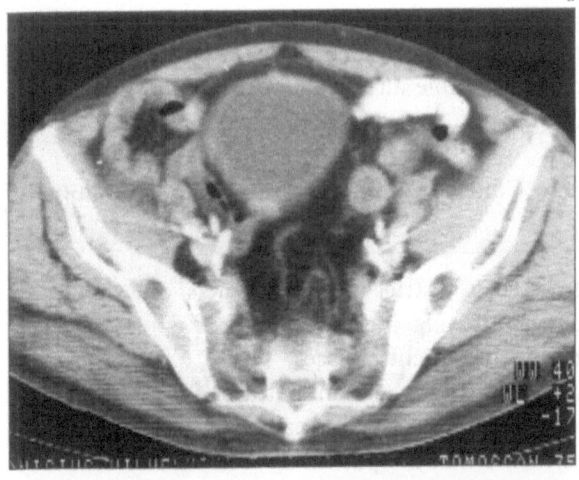
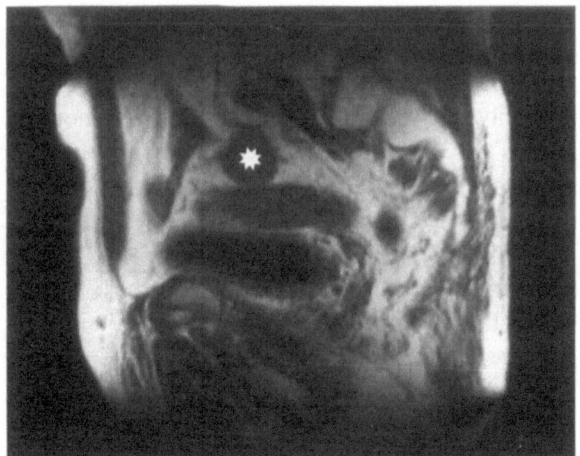
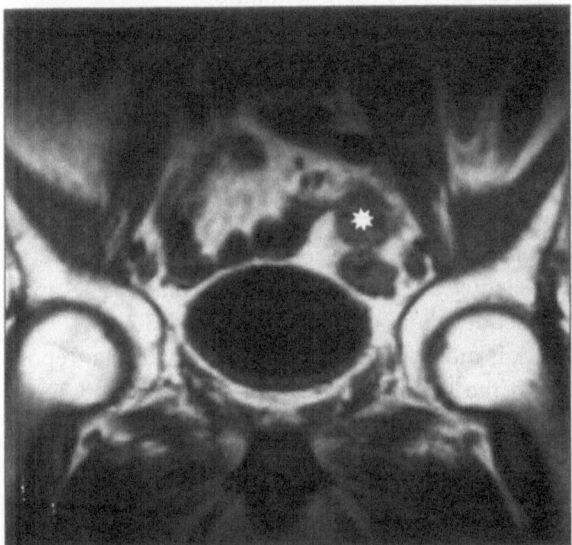
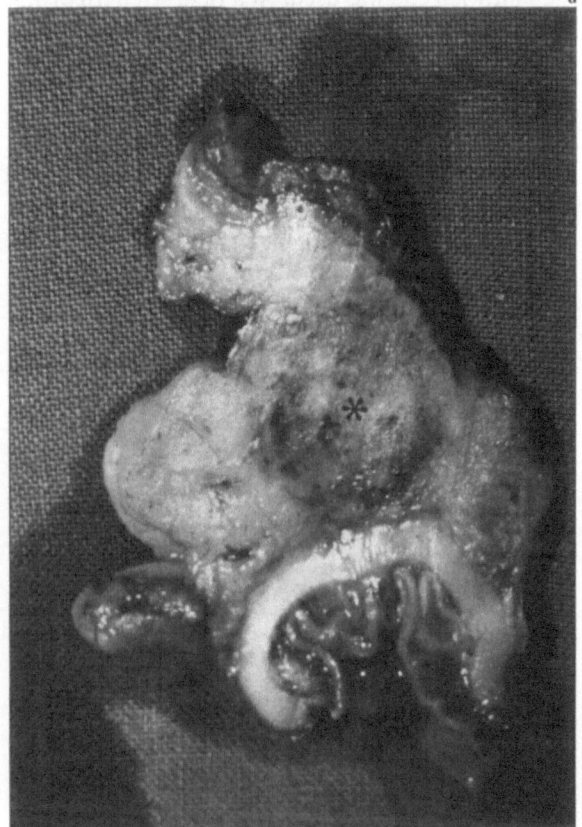

Fig. 3-22. Patient S. (a) The CT scan does not reveal any abnormalities. On MR images made in (b) the sagittal and (c) frontal planes (0.5 T; SE/750/30/2), a round tumor (*) can be seen just above a bowel loop. (d) Histologic examination revealed metastasis of the carcinoma of the urinary bladder, attached to a bowel loop.

The T-staging results obtained at 0.5 T with the sandwich coil were very reliable. If the T0-group is disregarded, at 0.5 T, incorrect staging results were obtained only in two patients. At 1.5 T, the tumors in stages Ta-T3A were often overstaged. The staging results for tumors in stages T3B and higher did not differ significantly at 0.5 T and 1.5 T.

Table 16 presents the staging results for the N stages. At 0.5 T, an incorrect normal result was obtained in 3 of the 15 patients. Furthermore, in 3 patients the technique failed to produce an adequate image of the high-iliac and para-aortic lymph nodes. This happened because the field of view was too small because the sandwich coil was used. At a field strength of 1.5 T, no incorrect results were found in any of the 43 patients.

A distant metastasis only was found in one of the patients (patient S.) examined at 0.5 T, in this case in the sigmoid colon (Fig. 3-22). The other distant metastases were found at 1.5 T. The larger area displayed probably has something to do with this.

3.5.3   Discussion

One has to be careful when making statements about differences in staging, because one is dealing with two separate groups of patients. Also, the number of patients examined at 0.5 T is small. Nevertheless, the results give an indication of the value of MRI at two field strengths in the staging of UBC.
The *T staging* at a field strength of 0.5 T (including sandwich coil) is slightly better for tumors in stages Ta-T2 than the staging at 1.5 T (without optimal surface coil). This can probably be explained by the very high signal-to-noise ratio (and thus the better image quality) that can be obtained with sandwich coil. If surface coils are not used, the signal-to-noise ratio at 1.5 T is better than that at 0.5 T.
The staging of the tumors in stages T3B or higher at a field strength of 0.5 T (with sandwich coil) is equal to that at 1.5 T (without surface coil).

The determination of *lymph node metastases* and *distant metastases* is clearly better at 1.5 T. This is due to the much larger field of view because of not using the sandwich coil. It is precisely the staging of tumors in stages T3A and higher and the establishment of metastases which are so important clinically. Accordingly, when staging UBC, preference is given

to MRI at a field strength of minimally 1.5 T, where the staging results can still be improved by using an optimal double surface coil with not too small a field of view.

3.6   Conclusion and the protocol to be followed

3.6.1.   Patient related factors

In order to restrict motion artifacts, one should:
a. keep the imaging time as short as possible,
b. put the patient at ease,
c. administer Buscopan® intravenously (0.5 ml) and intramuscularly (1.5 ml).
d. ensure that the patient does not eat or drink for 4 hours before the examination.
The urinary bladder should be neither too full nor too empty during the examination. This can be achieved by asking the patient to urinate 2 hr before the examination and then not until after completion.

3.6.2.   Optimal sequences

In order to assess the extent of UBC, several T_1-weighted SE images should be made. The optimal sequence, as found in section 3.3.3 (SE/750/15/2), is more or less in accordance with that reported in the literature (see Table 9). Only the TE is slightly shorter (15 ms). Because of the limitation of the MRI equipment, this study used the SE/750/30/2 sequence.

At least one T_2-weighted image also should be made. The sequence for this, determined in section 3.3.3 (SE/2100/100/2), is in agreement with the findings of other authors (see Table 9). In order to evaluate the mucous membrane of the urinary bladder, a proton-weighted image (SE/2100/30/2) can be made simultaneously with this T_2-weighted image. The STIR image appears to be valuable in showing lymph node and bone marrow metastases. The optimal sequence is IR/2000/225/ $\leq$ 60/2. This conforms with the experience of other authors.[44, 45, 61]

3.6.3.   Surface coils and strenght of the magnetic field

If a double surface coil with not too small a field of view is used, imaging and staging of UBC are improved.
For staging of UBC, MRI at a magnetic field strength of 1.5 T is preferable to 0.5 T.

IV

NORMAL MR IMAGES: CORRELATION WITH KWOWN ANATOMIC PROPORTIONS

4.1   Normal MR images of the pelvis

Before embarking on a discussion of MRI in carcinoma of the urinary bladder, it is essential to understand how to correlate the available anatomic topographic data with the MR images one acquires. In this chapter, we will do so by means of illustrations.

Section 4.1 presents a description of normal MR images of the male and female pelvis. In section 4.2, MR images and cross sections of anatomic material are correlated.

Finally, in section 4.3, MR images of a few cystectomy preparations are compared with the corresponding cross sections.

4.1.1   The male pelvis

In order to assess pelvic structures both T_1 and T_2 weighted images must be produced (see also section 3.3). The various organs (e.g., urinary bladder and lymph nodes) are easiest to distinguish on T_1-weighted images (Fig. 2-13), whereas the T_2-weighted images allow some discrimination between the various tissues. A survey of the signal intensities of the various tissues on these types of images is presented in Table 8. The next few sections will discuss the normal anatomic proportions of various pelvic structures, as seen on MR images.

Because the *urinary bladder*[75, 87, 95, 139, 219] is closely related to many surrounding organs, a proper assessment requires images to be made in at least three planes. The signal intensity of the normal urinary bladder wall is equal to that of muscle tissue, as the bladder largely consists of smooth muscle. On a T_1-weighted image, the wall of the urinary bladder has a slightly higher signal intensity than that of urine and a much lower signal intensity than that of perivesical fat. On T_2-weighted images, the contrast between urinary bladder wall and fat decreases. The contrast between urine and bladder wall, conversely increases on T_2-weighted images: the signal intensity of the bladder wall is lower than that of urine[34, 95, 106, 107] (Fig. 4-1).

Sometimes the mucosa is visible on a proton-weighted image as a thin high-intensity line. This is usually observed at the site of the urinary bladder floor (Figs. 4-2 and 4-5a). If this line is very obvious, then one is dealing with submucosal edema or mucosal hyperemia. On sagittal images, one can see the median umbilical ligament (remainder of the urachus) on the ventrocranial side of the bladder (Fig. 4-3). The plica interureterica is not usually visible on MR images. It can, however, be recognized on the MR image when there is hypertrophy of the urinary bladder wall (Fig. 4-17).

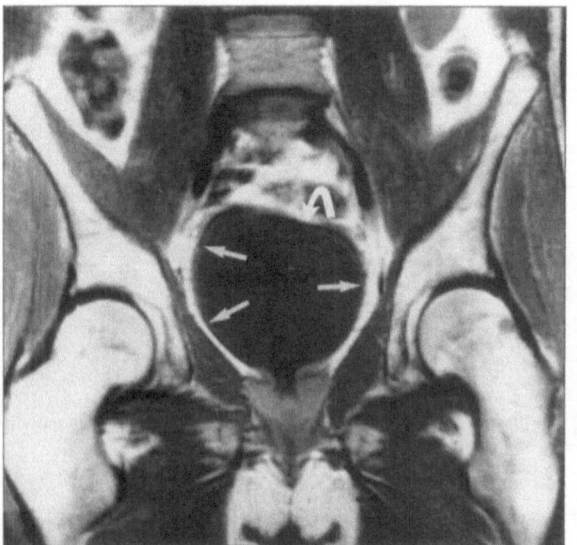 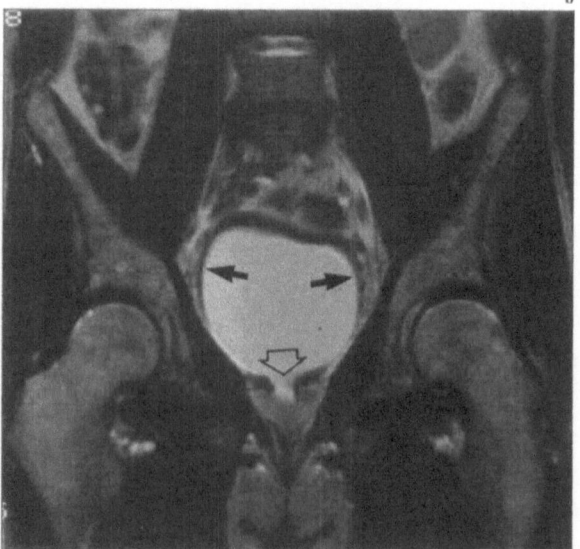

Fig. 4-1. (a) T1- weighted and **(b)** T2-weighted MR images in the coronal plane (1.5 T; SE/1000/15/2 and SE/2000/100/2). The gray thin bladder wall can hardly be recognized on the T1-weighted image (arrows). The contrast between bladder wall (solid black arrows) and urine is better on the T2-weighted image. The fat-shift artifact (curved arrow) does, however, have a disturbing effect. The wall is thicker around the neck of the bladder (open arrow).

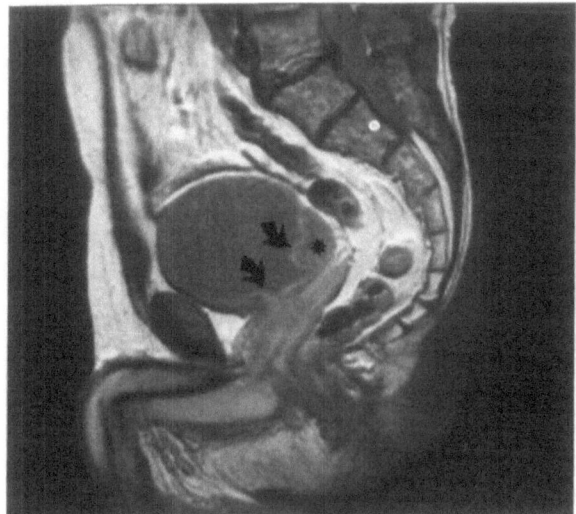

Fig. 4-2. Sagittal MR image with intermediate sequence (1.5 T; SE/2000/30/2). A thin white layer can be seen covering the tumor (*) and on the bladder floor (arrows), suggesting mucosal hyperemia or edema.

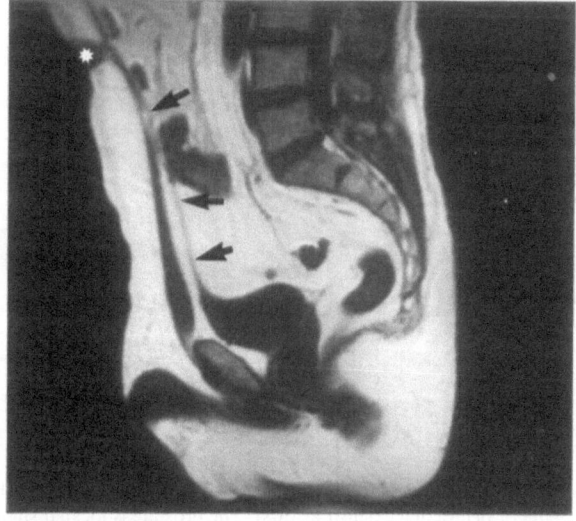

Fig. 4-3. A thin black line (arrows) can be seen on the sagittal MRI image (1.5 T; SE/700/30/2) between the navel (*) and the ventral side of the bladder. This is compatible with the location of the median umbilical ligament (remainder of the urachus).

The *ureters*[34, 79, 106, 107] are not usually visible. Sometimes they can be recognized as thin gray lines (Fig. 4-4). On dilatation they can be well delineated with a signal intensity similar to that of urine. In these situations, the preferred directions for imaging are coronal and transverse.

Muscles (iliopsoas, internal obturator, levator ani, gluteal, piriform, and transverse perineal) are well delineated on T_1- weighted images, which give the optimal contrast between muscle and fat (Fig. 2-13).[34, 106, 107]

T_1-weighted images are also the most suitable for imaging *lymph nodes*,[43, 57] as on these images, lymph nodes' signal intensity is lower than that of the surrounding fatty tissue. Images in the coronal and transverse planes are preferred to those in the sagittal plane. Nonpathologic, enlarged lymph nodes are difficult to identify (Fig. 4-4). The maximum length of a normal lymph node is 13 mm,[57] and the maximum diameter is 10 mm.[43]

Optimal imaging of the *prostate*[21, 175] requires images to be made in three planes. The best delineation of prostate from urinary bladder floor is achieved with the sagittal plane and a slightly angled coronal plane. As the prostate is located somewhat dorsal to the bladder floor, this angle ensures the perpendicu-

larity of the plane separating the two structures (Fig. 4-5).

On T_1-weighted images, the prostate has a homogeneous, fairly low signal intensity that is equal to that of muscle tissue (Fig. 4-5b). On sagittal images, the prostate can be readily distinguished from the rectum (Fig. 4-5a). T_2-weighted images are necessary to distinguish the prostate from the surrounding venous plexus. On these images, the prostate has a low signal intensity, whereas the venous plexus has a strong signal (Fig. 4-6).

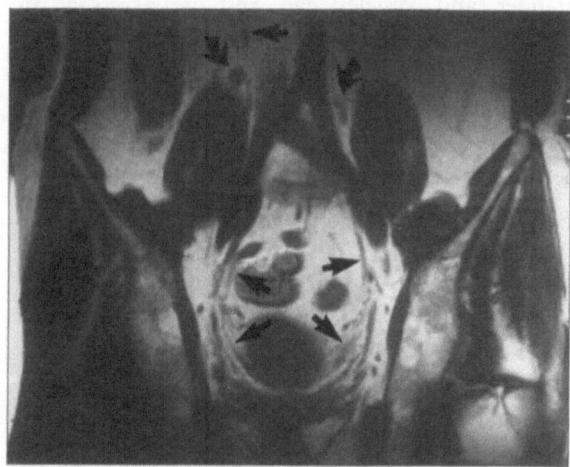

Fig. 4-4. On the coronal T1-weighted MR image (1.5 T; double surface coil; SE/650/30/2), the ureters can be traced as thin black lines as far as the bladder (straight arrows). Lymph nodes that are not quite enlarged also can be seen paracavally and paraaortic (curved arrows).

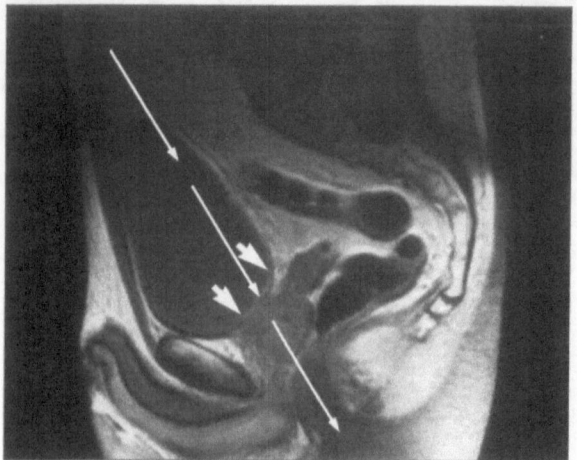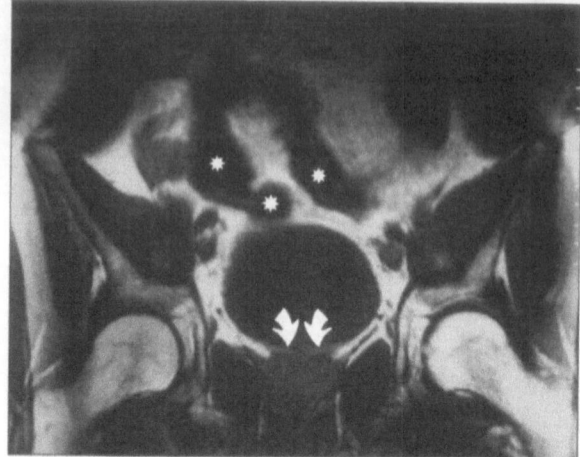

Fig. 4-5. (a) On the sagittal MR image (1.5 T; SE/2000/30/2), a thin clear line can be seen on the bladder floor, suggesting mucosal edema or hemorrhage (short arrows). The prostate is located slightly dorsal to the bladder floor. On the sagittal image, the prostate and seminal vesicles can be distinguished from the rectum. **(b)** On the angulated MR image (1.5 T; SE/750/30/4), the bladder floor can be distinguished from the prostate (curved arrows) thanks to a thin interposing fat layer. The angle is indicated on **(a)** (long arrows). There is a very close relationship between intestine (*) and bladder roof.

Between the urinary bladder lumen and the prostate, the muscle tissue of the bladder floor and the ostium can be recognized on T_2-weighted images (Figs. 4-1 and 4-6). The prostate capsule cannot always be distinguished.

On T_1-weighted images, the normal signal intensity of the *seminal vesicles*[79,95] resembles that of muscle tissue (Figs. 2-9, 4-7a, and 4-17a). The signal intensity on T_2-weighted images is high (Fig. 4-7b). The signal intensity of the seminal vesicles must be symmetrical (Figs. 2-9 and 4-6a). The plane separating bladder and vesicles can best be assessed on T_1-weighted images made in the transverse or sagittal planes. A thin, high-signal fat layer can be seen on these images between the vesicles and the bladder (Figs. 2-9, 4-5a, 4-17a, and 4-17b). The boundary between the seminal vesicles and the prostate can be seen on T_1-weighted images (Fig. 4-5a and 4-17b).

The *vasa deferens*[79,95] are best displayed on T_1-weighted images in the coronal plane. The vasa deferens can be recognized by their low signal intensity compared with that of the surrounding fatty tissue (Fig. 4-8).

Because of the high level of moisture, the corpora cavernosa and the corpus spongiosum of the *penis*[106,111] are clearly visible on T_2-weighted images. The corpus spongiosum has a higher signal intensity

than do the corpora cavernosa. One can usually recognize the urethra in the middle of the corpus spongiosum.

The *testicles*[204] show a homogeneous signal intensity equal to that of muscle tissue on T_1-weighted images. On T_2-weighted images, the signal intensity is high. The tunica albuginea consists of connective tissue and has a low signal intensity on both T_1- and T_2-weighted images.

Because of air in the lumen and the surrounding fatty tissue, the *intestines*[34,106,107] (particularly the rectosigmoid colon) are well delineated on T_1-weighted images. In order to assess the relationship between the bladder and the rectosigmoid colon, it is preferable to use images in the sagittal and transverse planes. The cecum and appendix are sometimes easy to recognize in obese patients. The ileum and the sigmoid colon may be closely related to the fundus of the urinary bladder (Figs. 2-13, 3-22, 4-5b, and 4-15a). The peritoneum is sometimes, although not always, recognizable as a layer of low signal intensity on both T_1- and T_2-weighted images (Fig. 4-15a). Differentiation between pathologically enlarged lymph nodes and intestines can prove difficult (Fig. 2-13). A suitable contrast medium for the intestine would facilitate this differentiation, but as yet, no such media are available. This subject will be dealt with in more detail in section 6.2 2.

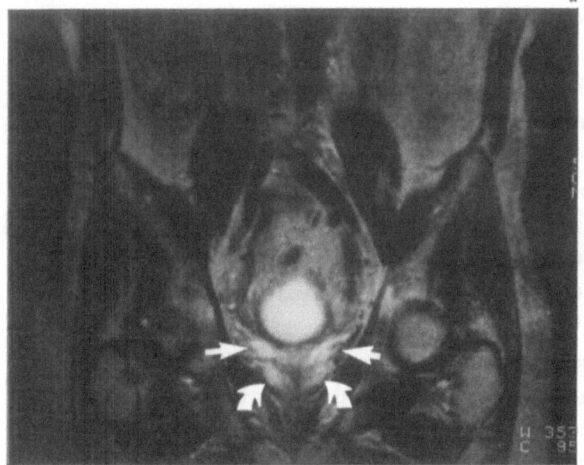
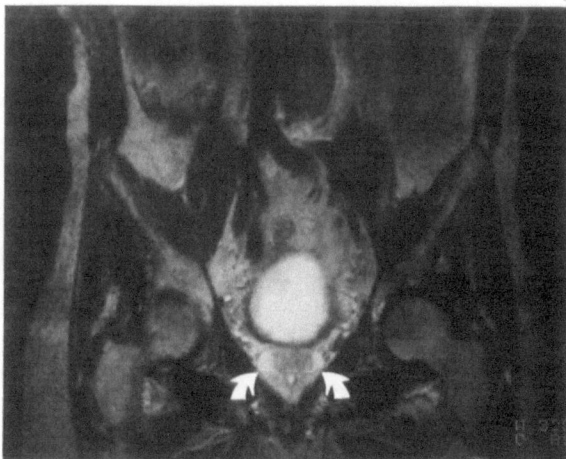
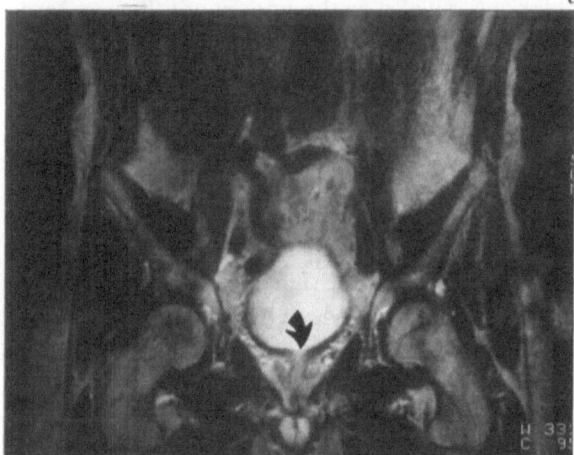

Fig. 4-6. Consecutive T2-weighted MR images in the coronal plane (1.5 T; SE/2000/1000/2). **(a)** The most dorsal slice: the seminal vesicles (straight arrows) and the venous plexus around the prostate (curved white arrows) can easily be recognized owing to their high signal intensity, **(b)** and **(c)**, More ventral slices: the prostate can be recognized centrally because of its lower signal intensity. The neck of the bladder (curved black arrow) can be distinguished by an interruption of the muscle layer on the bladder floor. The bladder wall can clearly be distinguished clearly from urine because of its lower signal intensity on all images.

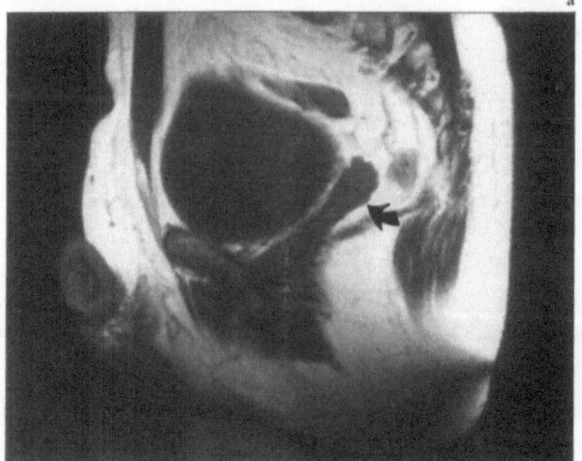
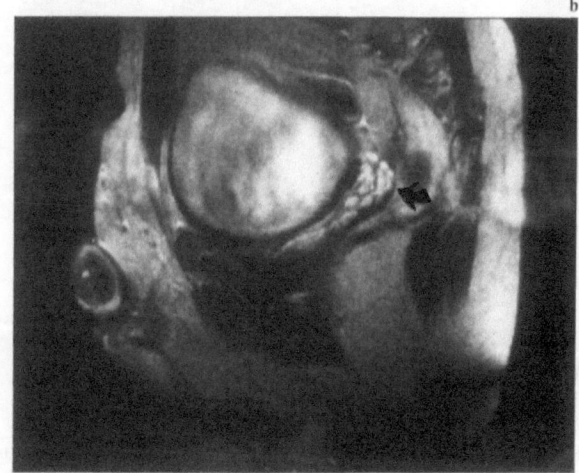

Fig. 4-7. Sagittal MR images. **(a)** On the T1-weighted image (1.5 T; SE/750/30/2) the seminal vesicles (arrow) have a signal intensity similar to that of muscle tissue. **(b)** On the T2-weighted image (1.5 T; SE/2000/100/2), they have a high signal intensity (arrow).

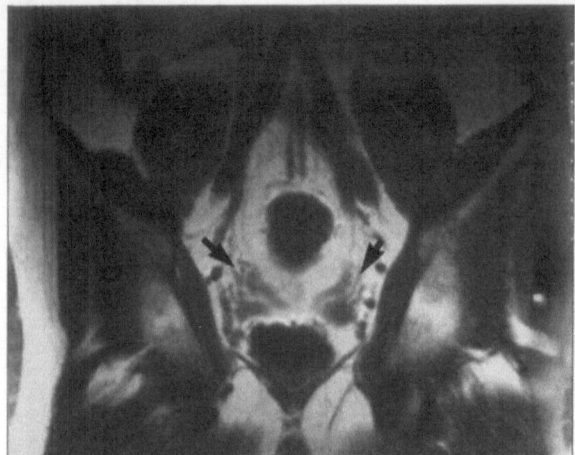

Fig. 4-8. The vasa deferens (arrows) can be seen on the coronal MR image (1.5 T; SE/750/30/2).

Because of the lack of signal ('flow-void' phenomenon)[12, 30] in the *large vessels*, these can be well distinguished from the intestines with all imaging sequences (Fig. 2-13).

As the presence of *bone marrow metastases* in patients with a UBC has far-reaching consequences for the choice of therapy, and because MRI seems to be a promising technique for detection of bone marrow metastases, the next section will consider in more detail the visualization of bone marrow by using MRI.[221]

Bone marrow is composed of a trabecular bone network, containing fat cells, hematopoietic cells, reticuloendothelial cells, nerve fibers and vascular sinu-

soids.[214] The variety and complexity of the various anatomic, physiologic, and biochemical structures in the bone marrow can be simplified by dividing bone marrow into two types: red, hematopoietic, active bone marrow, and yellow, hematopoietic, inactive bone marrow. The latter mainly consists of fat cells.

In adults, red marrow is largely found in the axial skeleton, the skull, the proximal humeri and proximal femurs. As age increases, a conversion of red to yellow bone marrow occurs: the volume of red bone marrow in the vertebral bodies decreases from 58% to 29% in the eight decade of life.[60] The MRI signal does not depend only on the concentration of trabecular bone, but also on the amount of yellow and red marrow. The fat-rich, yellow bone marrow produces a high signal on T_1-weighted images and an intermediate signal on T_2-weighted images. The signal intensity of red bone marrow is not as high on T_1-weighted images, whereas the signal on T_2-weighted images depends on the amounts of fat, water, and protein present.[221]

With increasing age, the signal intensity of the bone marrow increases on T_1-weighted images because of a decrease in the amount of red marrow and an increase in the amount of yellow marrow.[221] Cortical bone can be recognized on all images as the layer producing a poor signal around the marrow.[221]

4.1.2   The female pelvis

On T_1-weighted images, normal *ovaries*[42, 58, 110] have

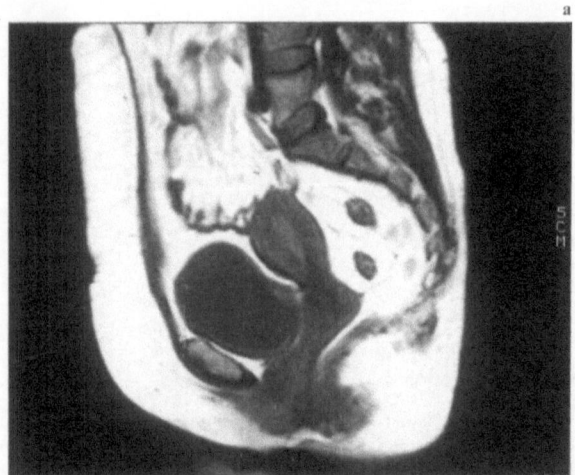
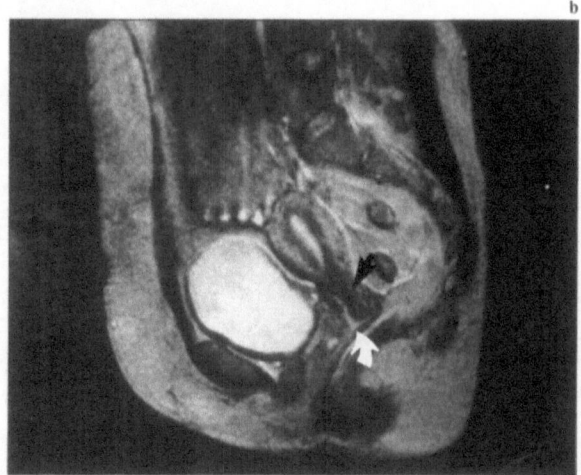

Fig. 4-9. Sagittal MR images. **(a)** Good demarcation between uterus and bladder roof on the T1-weighted image (1.5 T; SE/800/30/2) is due to the thin interposing layer of fat. **(b)** On the T2-weighted image (1.5 T; SE/2000/100/2), the various zones of the uterine wall can be distinguished. The low-signal cervical fibrous stroma (straight arrow) containing the centrally located high-signal cervical mucus (curved arrow) also can be recognized.

a

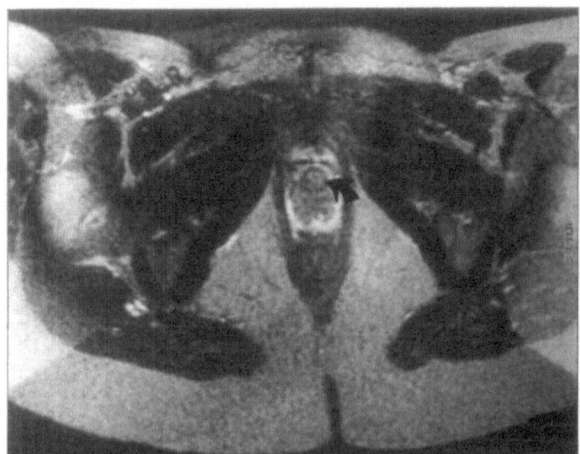

b

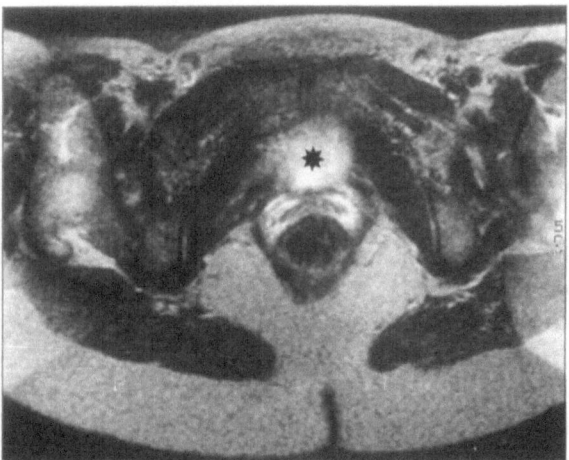

c

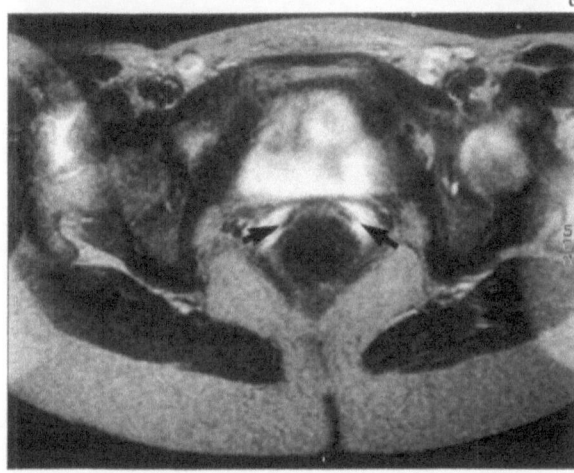

Fig. 4-10. Transverse MR images (1.5 T; SE/2000/100/2). **(a)** On the image taken through the bottom third of the vagina, the urethra can be seen ventral to the vagina (curved arrow). **(b)** The bladder (*) is situated ventral to the middle third of the vagina. **(c)** The uppermost third of the vagina is formed by the fornices (arrows).

- the peripheral layer of the myometrium has an intermediate signal intensity.

The MR image of the uterus is dependent on the menstrual cycle: during the secretory phase, the uterus is larger, the endometrium thicker, and the signal intensity of the myometrium is certainly low, but is nevertheless higher than it is in the proliferative phase.[94, 153]

The *cervix*[109, 110] is also best displayed on T_2-weighted images in the sagittal and transverse planes. On these images, there is a central area with high signal intensity: the endocervical mucus. The low-signal cervical fibrous stroma is located around this (Fig. 4-9b). The paracervical tissue has a signal intensity, both on T_1- and on T_2-weighted images, that resembles that of smooth muscle. Thus, paracervical tissue can be delineated from the fibrous stroma (on T_2-weighted images) and from the surrounding fatty tissue (on T_1-weighted images).

The *vagina*[48] is most clearly visible on T_2-weighted images in the transverse and sagittal planes. The anatomic division of the vagina into three parts (uppermost, middle, and bottom third) is well demonstrated on the transverse images:

- ventral to the bottom third, one can see the urethra (Fig. 4-10a),
- the urinary bladder is situated ventral to the middle third (Fig. 4-10b),

a signal intensity equal to that of muscle tissue. Distinguishing the ovaries from bowel loops can be difficult on these images. The vessels around the ovaries can be useful in aiding their detection. The ovaries' signal intensity on T_2-weighted images is similar to that of the surrounding fat. In the majority of women, the ovaries can be distinguished on MR images.[110] The diameter ranges from 1.5 to 2.5 cm. Either the transverse or the coronal plane is best for generating the image.

On T_1-weighted images, the *uterus*[55, 94, 109, 110, 112, 153] has a homogeneous signal intensity equal to that of muscle tissue (Fig. 4-9a). The various zones of the uterine wall can best be distinguished on T_2-weighted images in the sagittal and transverse planes (Fig. 4-9b):

- the high-signal endometrium is located centrally,
- the basal layer of the myometrium ('junctional zone') has a low signal intensity; this zone, however,cannot be recognized in the premenarchal or postmenopausal periods,

the uppermost third is formed by the fornices (Fig. 4-10c).

The signal intensities of the various parts of the vagina on T_2-weighted images also are dependent on the menstrual cycle. During the midsecretory phase, the vaginal wall has an intermediate signal intensity. Here, the central layer of mucus is thick and its signal is strong. During the early-proliferative and late-secretory phases, the wall has a poor signal and the central layer of mucus is much thinner. Thus, the optimal contrast is present in the early-proliferative and late-secretory phases. In women who have reached menopause or who are taking oral contraceptives, the vaginal wall produces a low signal and the central layer of mucus very thin (Fig. 4-10).

The fat layer between uterus in anteflexion of the vagina and bladder can be seen as a thin, high-signal layer on sagittal T_1-weighted images (Fig. 4-9).

4.2   Correlation of MR images with anatomic sections

Thanks to the unique and variable contrast between tissues, and the potential to acquire images in many planes, MRI can produce very accurate pictures of the true anatomy. In order to illustrate this and to increase insight into the technique of generating images, MR images of an anatomic specimen were prepared. For this purpose, a specimen of the lower abdomen and pelvis was frozen to -40°C. When the specimen was completely thawed out, T_1- and T_2-weighted images were produced in the sagittal plane. The slice thickness used for the MR images was 8 mm, the interslice interval was 1 mm. The preparation was then refrozen to -40°C, after which it could be sawed into thin, 9-mm slices, in keeping with the sagittal MR images. The correlation between MR images and crosssections is illustrated in Figures 4-11 to 4- 14. It is noticeable that muscles on the T_1- and T_2-weighted images have an abnormally high signal intensity. This could well be a postmortem effect (reduction of T_1 or prolongation of T_2). Furthermore, the large vessels in this specimen no longer give a low signal on the MR images, because of the lack of a flow-void phenomenon (see also section 4.1.2).

Fig. 4-11. Anatomic correlation between **(a)** cryosections and **(c)** T1-weighted (1.5 T; SE/800/30/2) and **(d)** T2-weighted (1.5 T; SE/2000/100/2) MR images. Image 4 cm left of the median line; slice thickness is 9 mm.

1. M. rectus abdominis
2. pubic bone/symphysis
3. M. pectineus
4. M. gluteus maximus
5. M. levator ani
6. internal iliac vessels
7. inferior mesenteric vessels
8. small-bowel loops
9. mesentery
10. common iliac artery
11. common iliac vein
12. rectum plug
13. rectum
14. sigmoid colon
15. ascending/transverse colon
16. peritoneum
17. urinary bladder
18. plica interureterica
19. prostate
20. seminal vesicles
21. plexus venosus vesicalis/prostatica
22. corpus cavernosum
23. corpus spongiosum
24. testicle
25. plexus venosus vertebrales interni

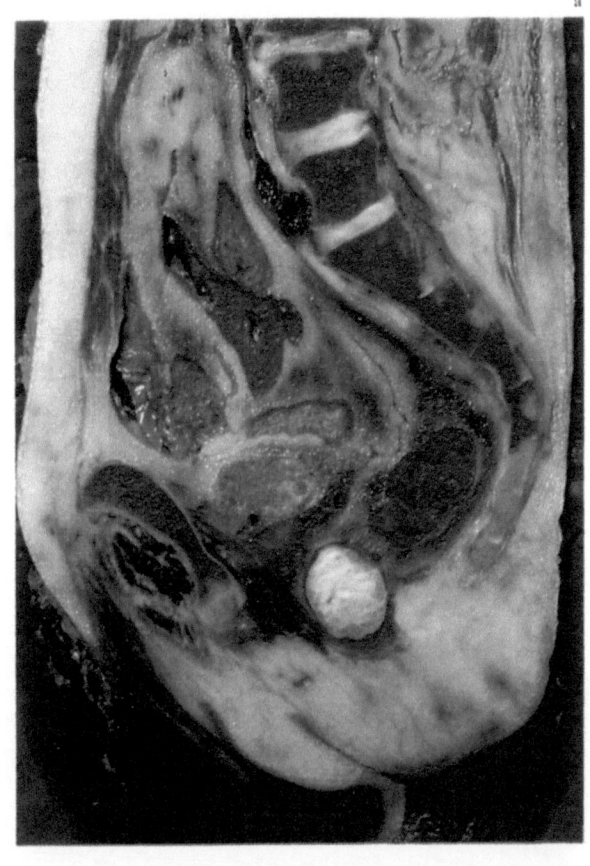

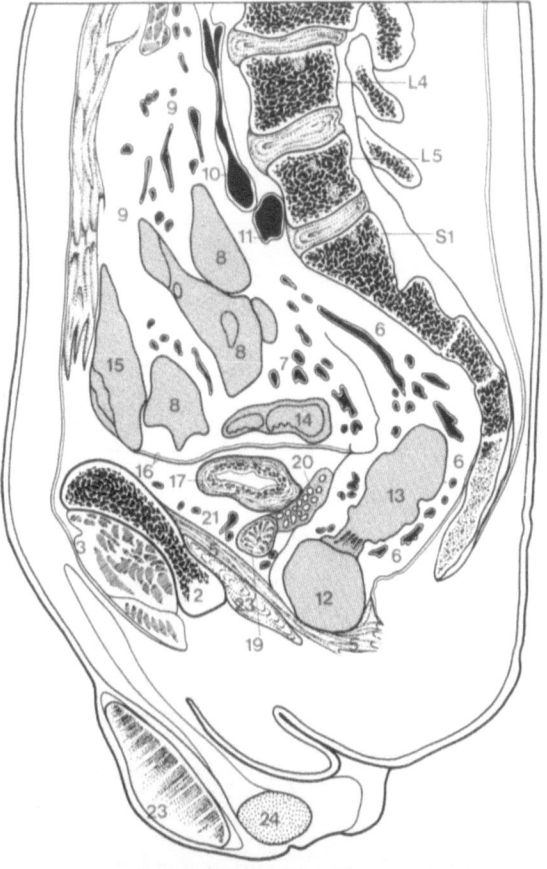

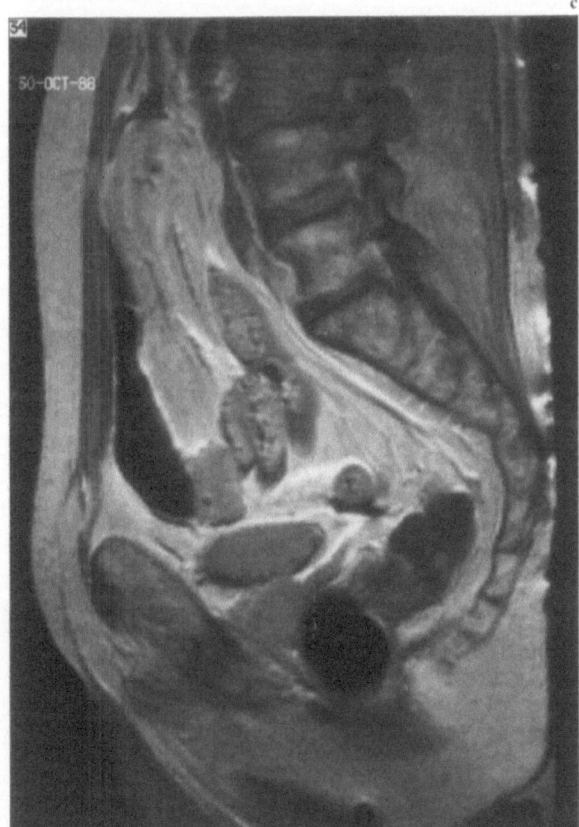

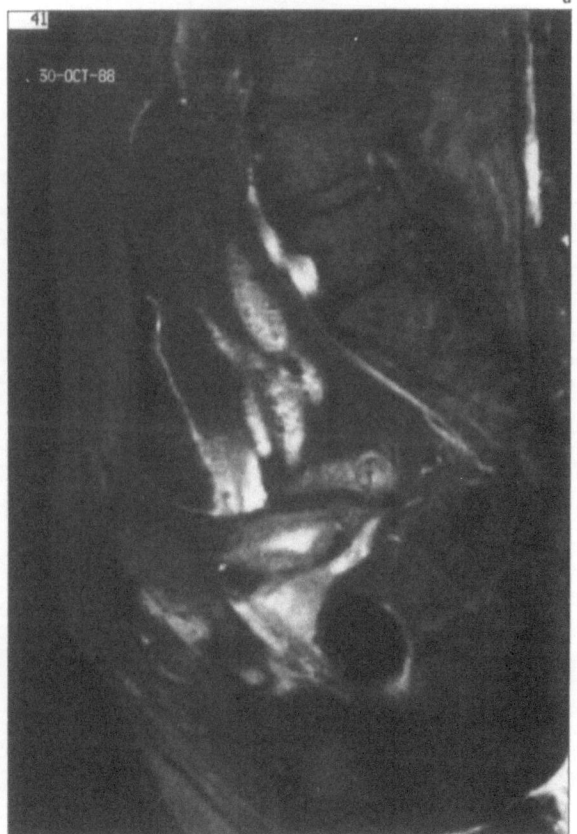

Fig. 4-12. Anatomic correlation between **(a)** cryosection and **(c)** T1-weighted (1.5 T; SE/800/30/2) and **(d)** T2-weighed (1.5 T; SE/2000/100/2) MR images. Image 2 cm left of the median line; slice thickness is 9 mm.

1. M. rectus abdominis
2. pubic bone/symphysis
3. M. pectineus
4. M. gluteus maximus
5. M. levator ani
6. internal iliac vessels
7. inferior mesenteric vessels
8. small-bowel loops
9. mesentery
10. common iliac artery
11. common iliac vein
12. rectum plug
13. rectum
14. sigmoid colon
15. ascending/transverse colon
16. peritoneum
17. urinary bladder
18. plica interureterica
19. prostate
20. seminal vesicles
21. plexus venosus vesicalis/prostatica
22. corpus cavernosum
23. corpus spongiosum
24. testicle
25. plexus venosus vertebrales interni

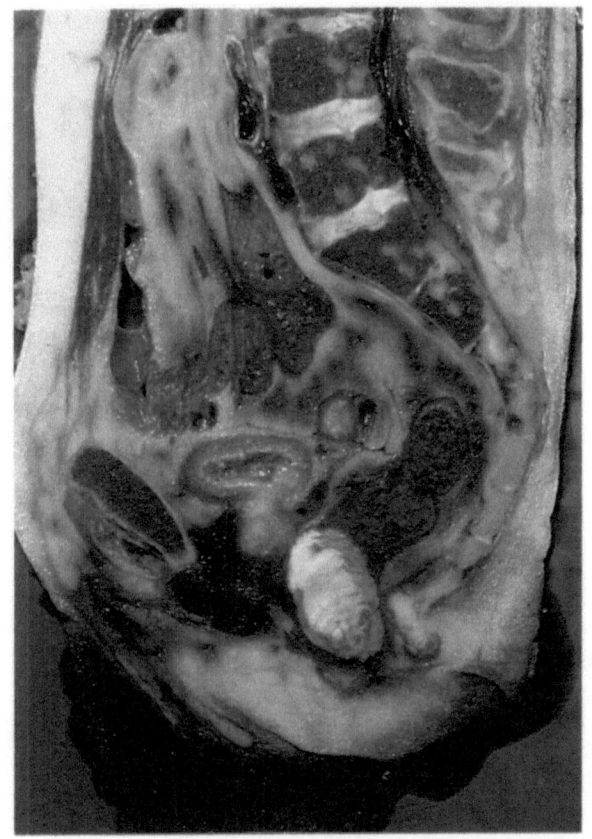

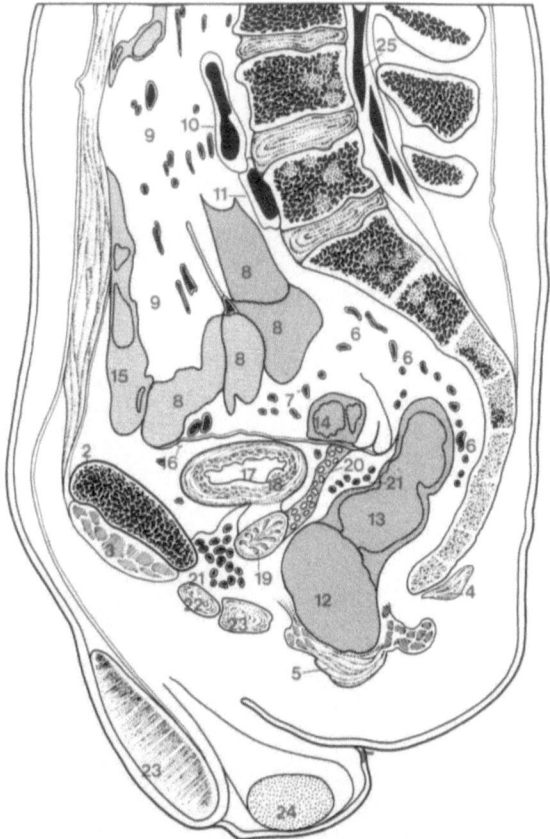

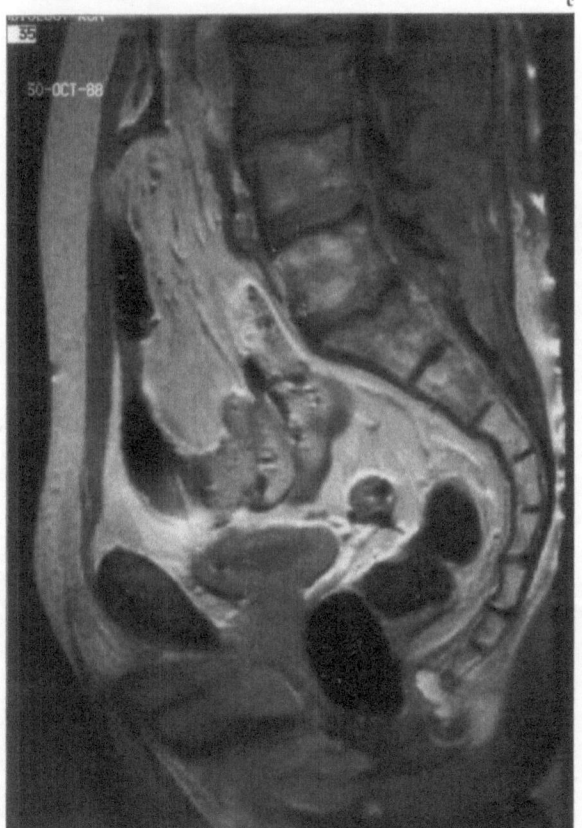

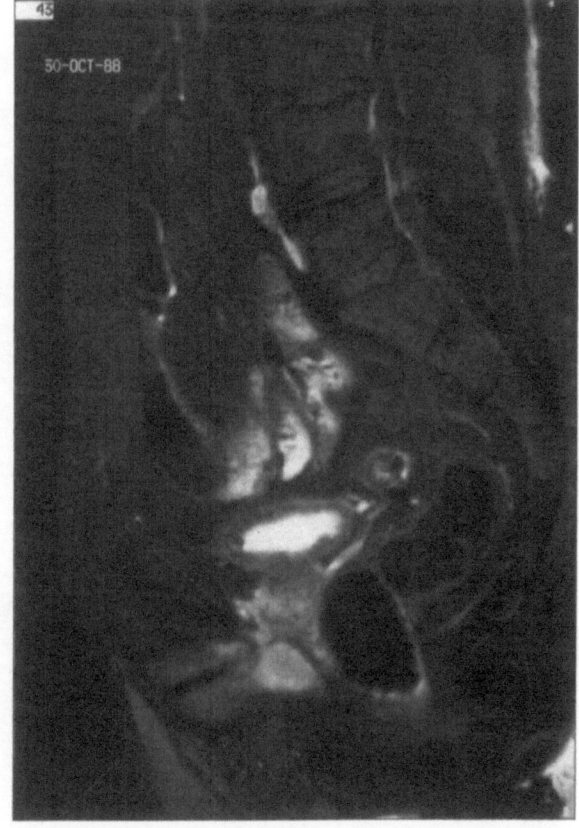

Fig. 4-13. Anatomic correlation between **(a)** cryosection and **(c)** T1-weighted (1.5 T; SE/800/30/2) and **(d)** T2-weighted (1.5 T; SE/2000/100/2) MR images. Image in the median line; slice thickness is 9 mm.

1. M. rectus abdominis
2. pubic bone/symphysis
3. M. pectineus
4. M. gluteus maximus
5. M. levator ani
6. internal iliac vessels
7. inferior mesenteric vessels
8. small-bowel loops
9. mesentery
10. common iliac artery
11. common iliac vein
12. rectum plug
13. rectum
14. sigmoid colon
15. ascending/transverse colon
16. peritoneum
17. urinary bladder
18. plica interureterica
19. prostate
20. seminal vesicles
21. plexus venosus vesicalis/prostatica
22. corpus cavernosum
23. corpus spongiosum
24. testicle
25. plexus venosus vertebrales interni

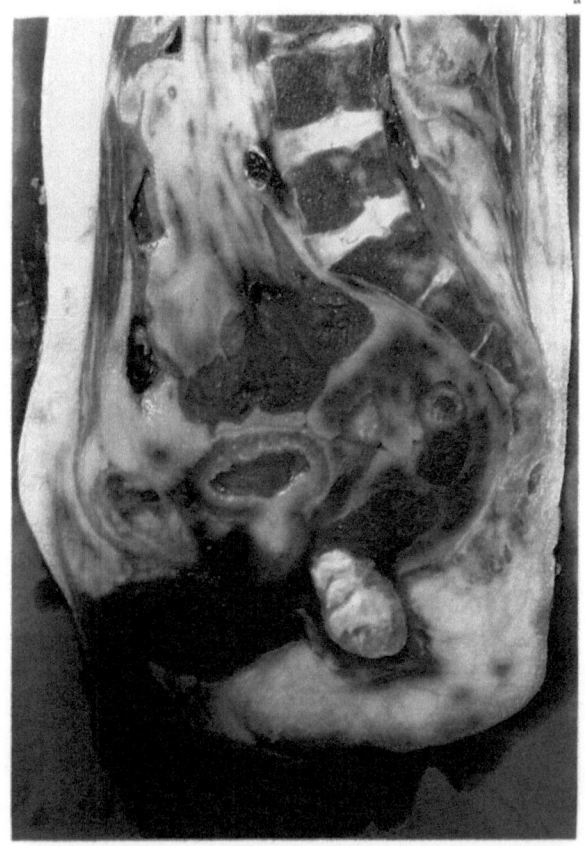
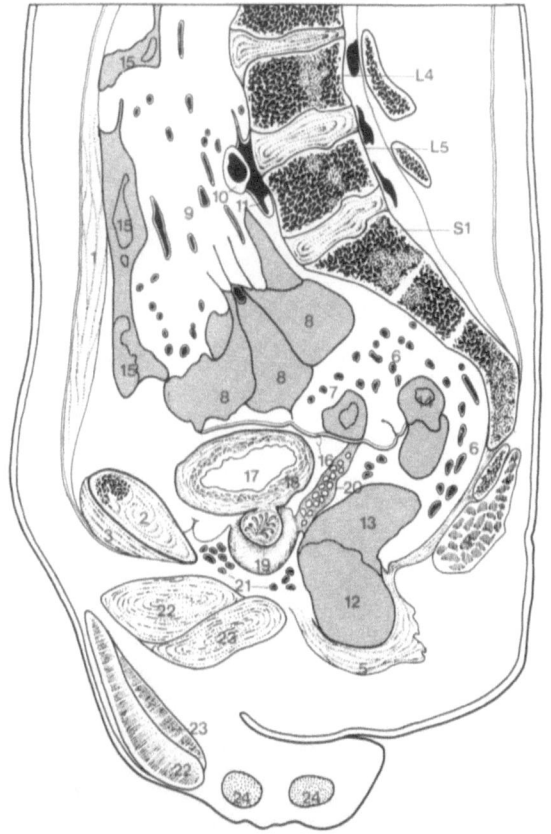
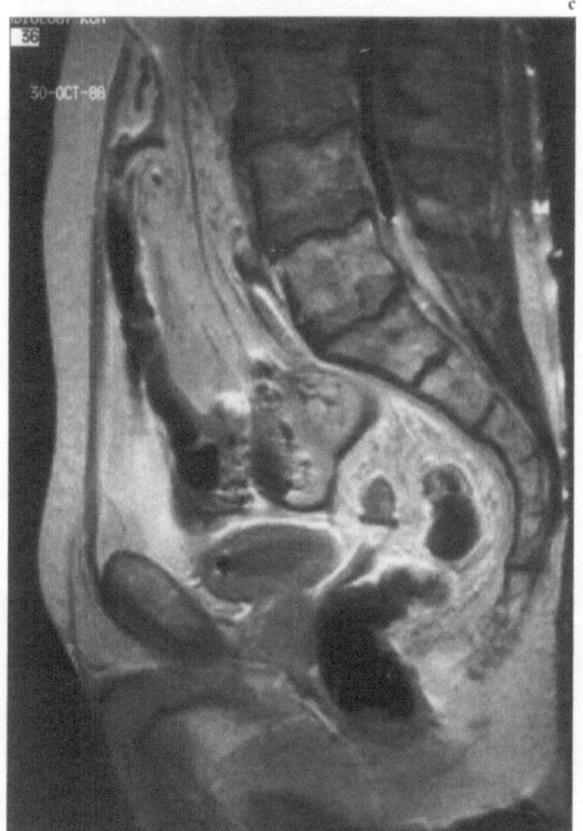
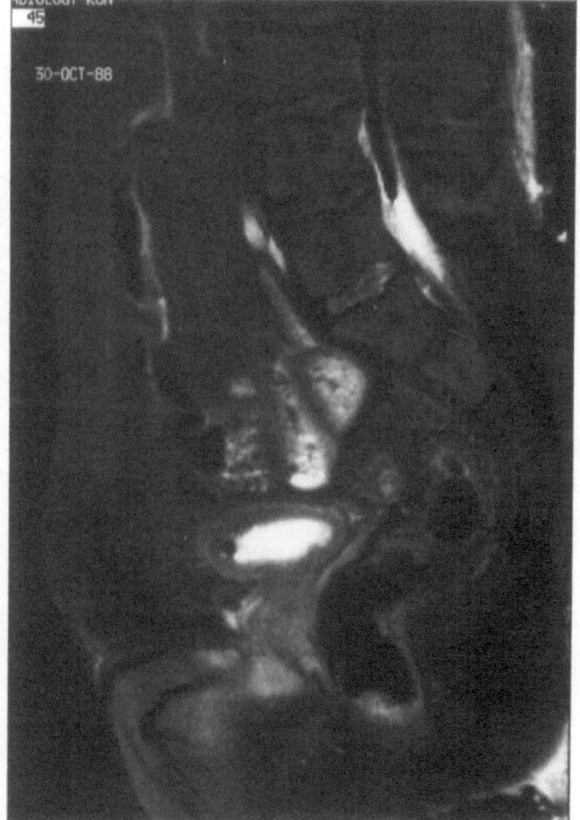

Fig. 4-14. Anatomical correlation between **(a)** cryosection and **(c)** T1-weighted (1.5 T; SE/800/30/2) and **(d)** T2-weighted (1.5 T; SE/2000/100/2) MR images. Image 2 cm right of the median line; slice thickness is 9 mm.

1. M. rectus abdominis
2. pubic bone/symphysis
3. M. pectineus
4. M. gluteus maximus
5. M. levator ani
6. internal iliac vessels
7. inferior mesenteric vessels
8. small-bowel loops
9. mesentery
10. common iliac artery
11. common iliac vein
12. rectum plug
13. rectum
14. sigmoid colon
15. ascending/transverse colon
16. peritoneum
17. urinary bladder
18. plica interureterica
19. prostate
20. seminal vesicles
21. plexus venosus vesicalis/prostatica
22. corpus cavernosum
23. corpus spongiosum
24. testicle
25. plexus venosus vertebrales interni

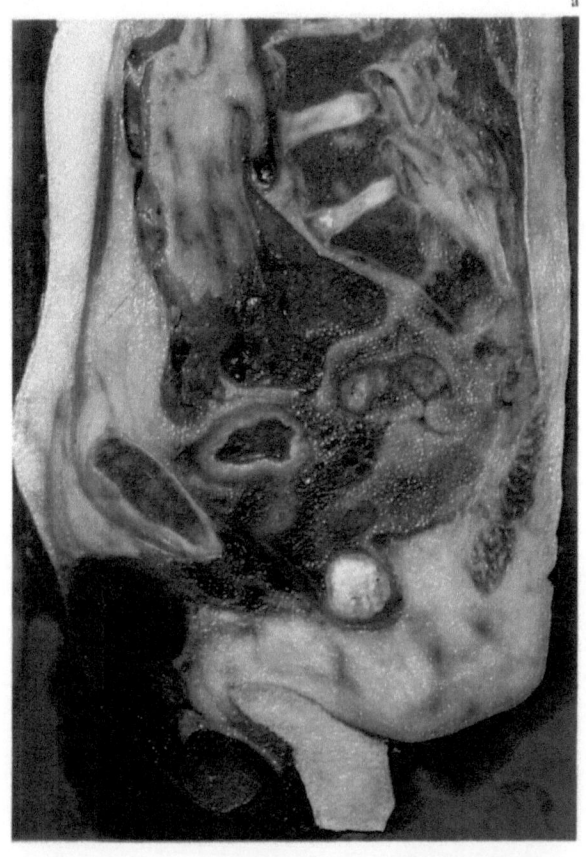
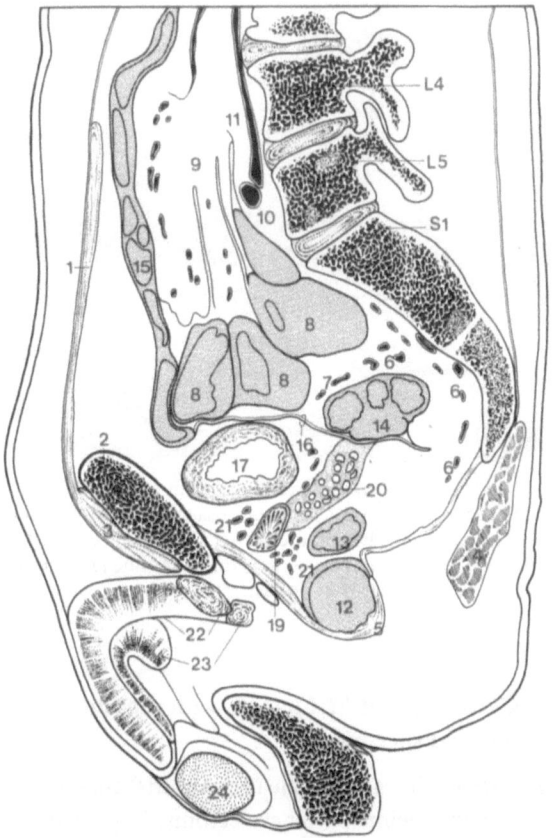
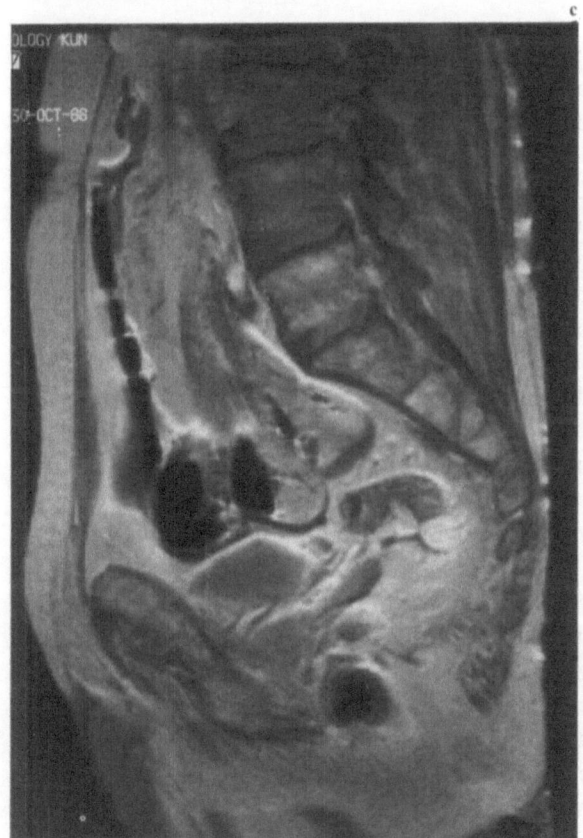
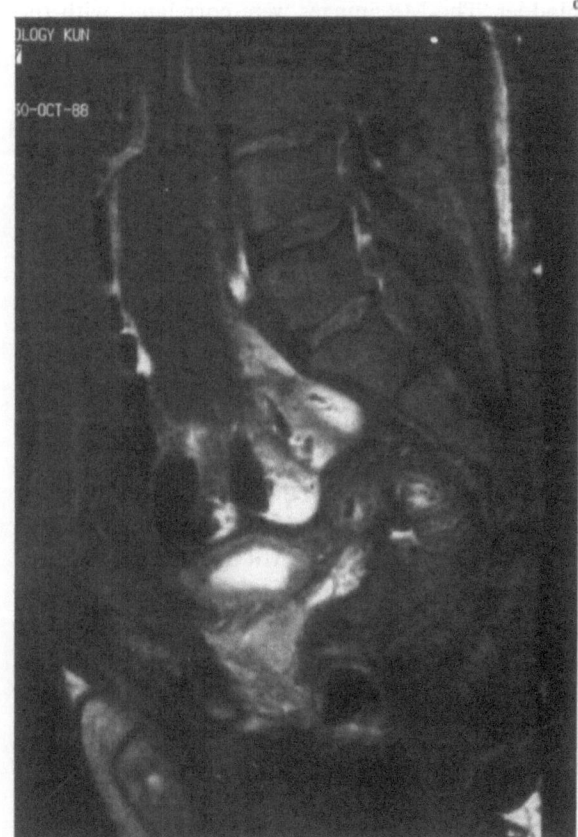

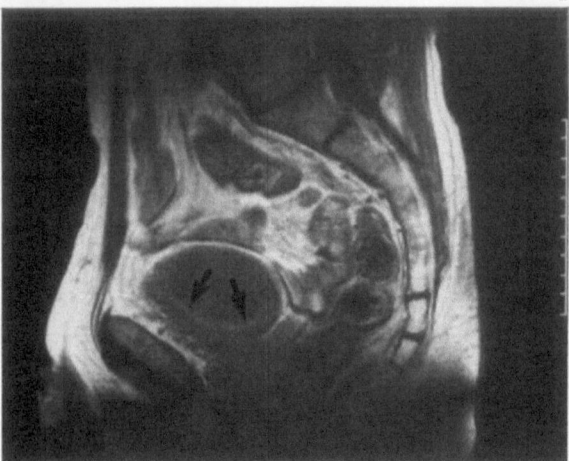

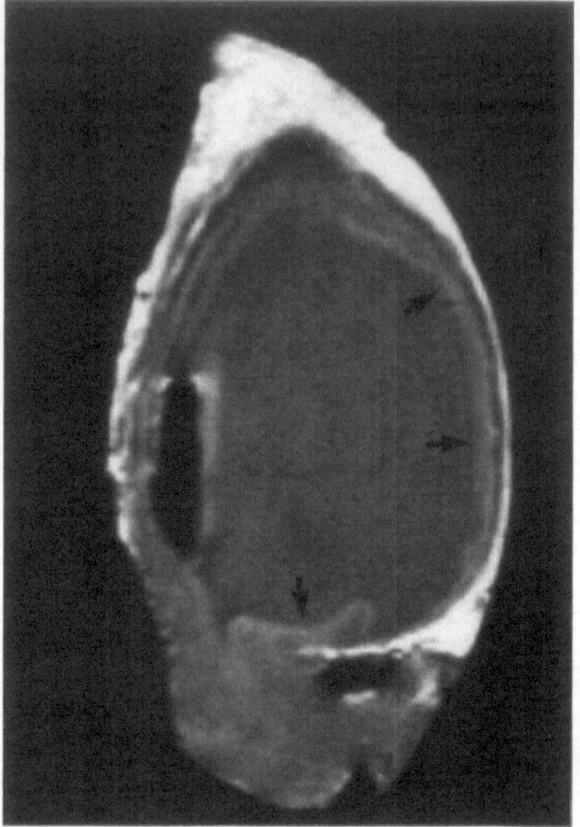

Fig. 4-15. On both the **(a)** in vivo and the **(b)** in vitro MR images (1.5 T; SE/850/30/2), the thickened mucosa can be seen as a thin clear layer (arrows). There is a close relationship between the intestine and the bladder. The peritoneum cannot be recognized easily because of the fat-shift artifact.

4.3 Correlation of MR images with sections resected specimens

In 11 patients it was possible to make MR images of the resected specimen after cystectomy. The purpose was to gain insight into the anatomy of the urinary bladder. The MR images were correlated with the macroscopic and histopathologic data on the resected specimens. Nine resected specimens were obtained from male patients, from whom the prostate and the seminal vesicles also were removed. The other two resected specimens were from female patients from whom both the urinary bladder and the uterus were removed.

The MRI examination was performed within 48 hours of the cystectomy. During the intervening period, the specimen was stored with the bladder empty at 4°C. For imaging, the specimen was placed in a hollow container. The urethra was sutured around a urinary bladder catheter. The bladder was then filled via this catheter with 250-300 ml physiologic saline. Then T_1- and T_2- weighted MR images were made in various directions. After the MRI study, the bladder was filled over a period of 24 hours with 250- 300 ml of 5% formaldehyde solution. One specimen, however, was filled with water and frozen. Once the macroscopic image of the resected specimen had been established photographically, a microscopic study was performed. In three specimens, no remnants of tumor were found during the histologic exa-

mination. The findings in these three patients are presented next. Findings in the other patients will be discussed in section 5.2.

On both T_1- and T_2-weighted images, the signal intensities of mucosa and urinary bladder wall of the resected specimen were higher than they had been before cystectomy. These findings agree with those of the anatomic material, as described in section 4.2. Presumably, this increased signal intensity is also due to a postmortem effect - a reduction in T_1 and/or a prolongation of T_2. There is no consensus in the literature on this point.[28] Therefore, it is not possible to obtain an exact correlation between in vivo and in vitro relaxation times.

Nevertheless, the MR images provided an excellent insight into the anatomy of the bladder: the bladder wall consists of four layers: the mucosa, the submucosa, the muscle layer, and the serosa. The serosa is absent in the region of the trigone (trigonum vesicae). The muscle layer consists of bundles of smooth muscle tissue and is sometimes called the detrusor urinae. At the site of the trigone, the wall also con-

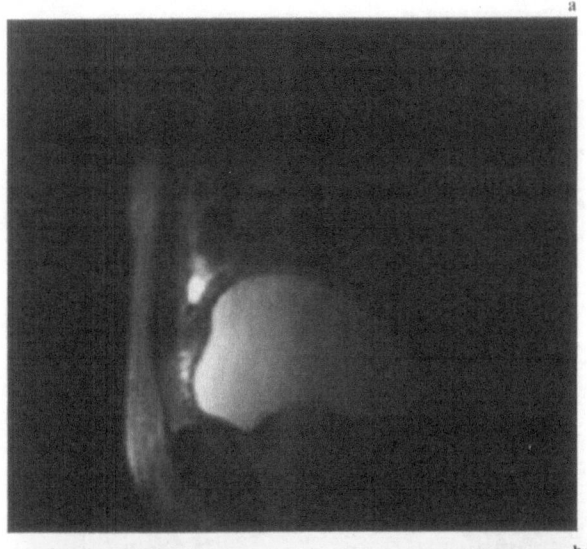

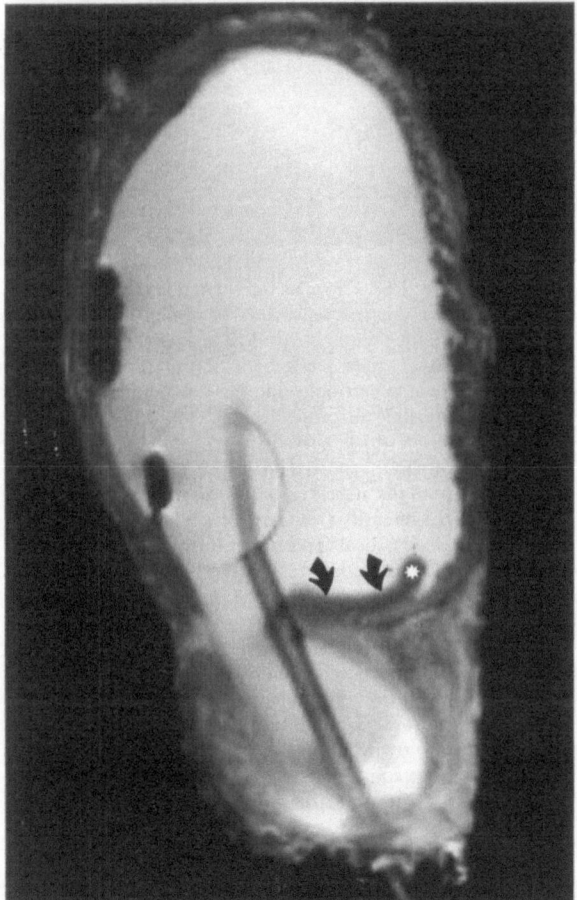

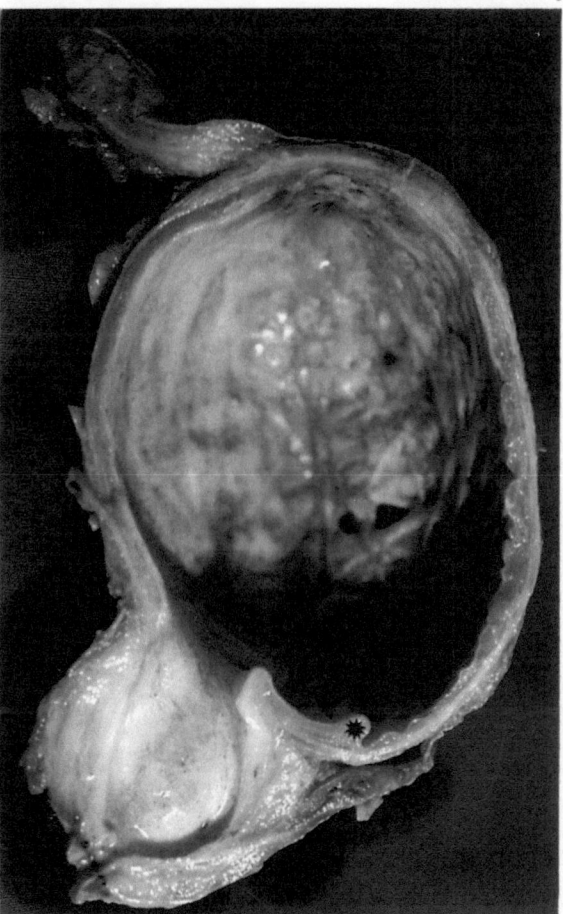

Fig. 4-16. The plica interureterica cannot be seen on **(a)** the in vivo MR image (1.5 T; SE/2000/100/2). It is visible on **(b)** the in vitro MR image (same parameters) and on **(c)** the resected specimen (*). Also, the thickened muscle layer at the site of the trigone can be seen on **(b)** as a low-signal layer (arrows), and also on **(c)**.

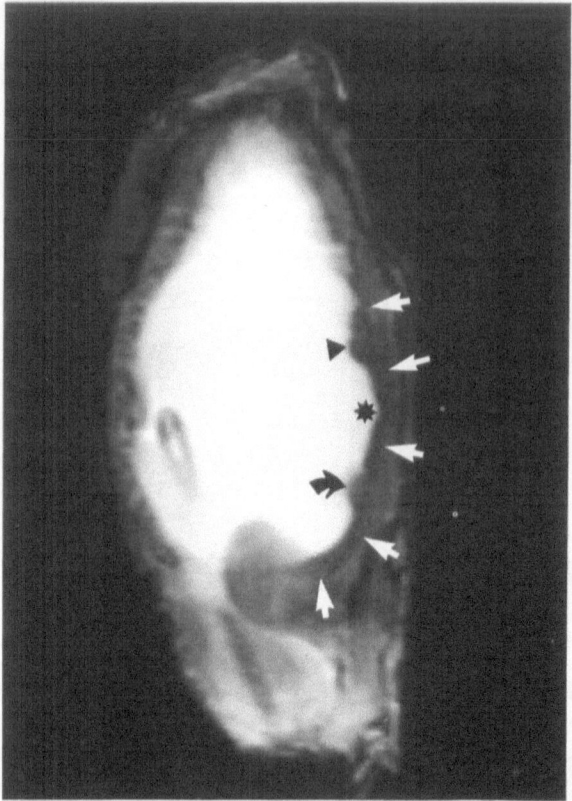

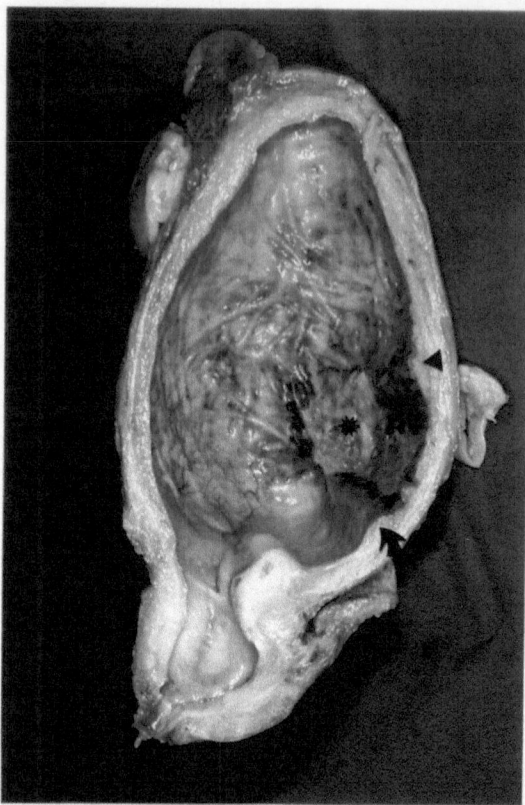

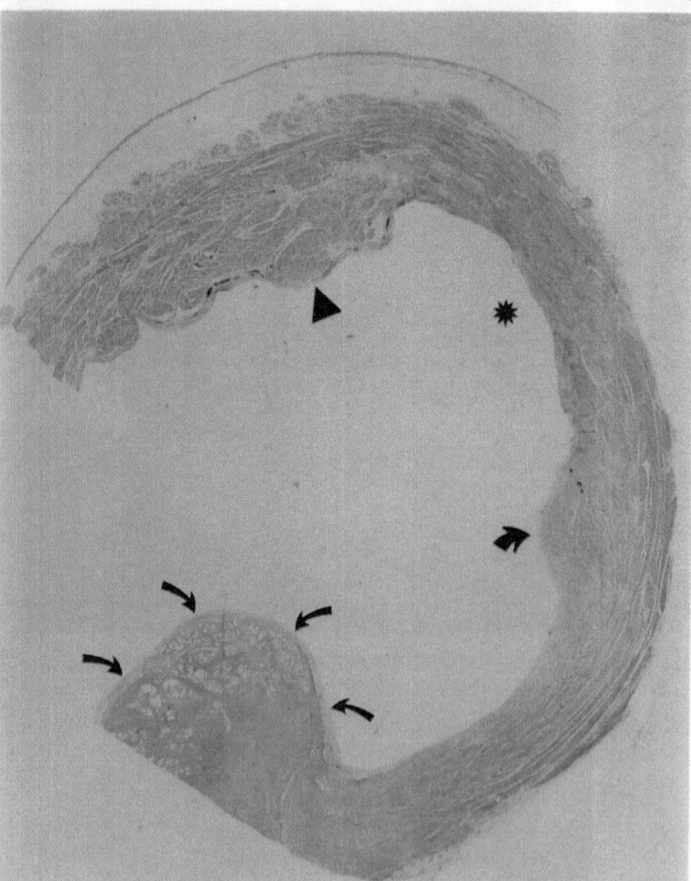

Fig. 4-17. The plica interureterica can be recognized (thick curved arrows) on **(d)** the transverse and **(e)** the sagittal in vivo MR images (1.5 T; SE/800/30/2). As a result of a transurethral resection, local hypertrophy and fibrous/granulation tissue is visible (arrowhead) cranial to the plica interureterica (thick, curved arrow).

(a) On the in vitro image (1.5 T; SE/2000/100/2), both the muscle layer and this area have a low signal intensity (white arrows). Plica (thick, curved arrow), local hypertrophy (arrowhead) and defect of transurethral resection (*) also can be seen on **(b)** the resected specimen and on **(c)** the microscopic image.

There is hypertrophy of the medial lobe of the prostate; because of this, the muscle layer over the prostate (see **(c)** microscopic image, thin, curved arrows) is very thin and hence invisible on both the in vitro MR image and the photograph of the resected specimen.

As a result of the prostate hypertrophy, there is also increased trabeculation of the bladder wall. The seminal vesicles (V), prostate (P) and rectum (R) are easily distinguished on the sagittal MR image **(e)**.

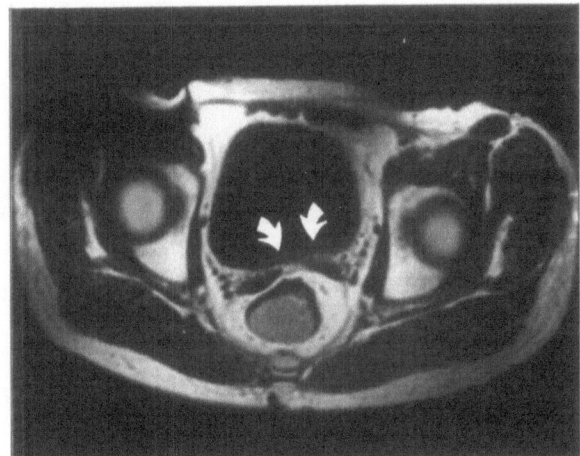

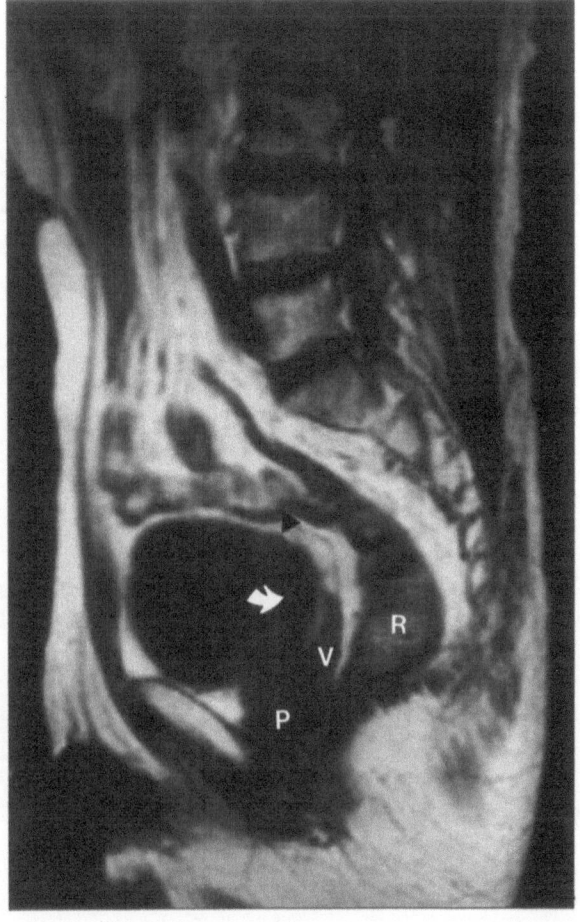

sists of a triangular layer of muscle, between the mucosa and the detrusor muscle. Bundles of this layer link the two ostia of the ureters, forming the plica interureterica, and there is an extra thickening in the median line of the muscle: the uvula. The bladder muscle layer is also often swollen at the front and on the bottom (Fig. 4-15a).

The serosa consists of a thin layer. Cranially and craniodorsally, this contains peritoneum; elsewhere it consists of connective tissue. The serosa is too thin to be recognized. Sometimes the fat-shift artifact (see section 2.5) is mistaken for the serosa (Fig. 4-15b).

The mucosa can sometimes be distinguished from the muscle layer, because the latter has a far higher signal intensity (Fig. 4-15).

The extra muscle layer at the site of the trigone (Fig. 4-16c) is easily seen on the in vitro MR images (Fig. 4-16b). The plica interureterica also can be clearly distinguished on in vitro MR images, unlike the situation on in vivo images (Fig. 4-16a). If the plica interureterica is visible on in vivo images, then this is indicative of bladder wall hypertrophy (trabeculated bladder) (Fig. 4-17).

The thin layer of muscle between the prostate and the urinary bladder lumen usually can be seen. However, if there is hypertrophy of the prostate (especially of the medial lobe), this layer can become extremely thin, and it may then no longer be distinguishable even on the images of the bladder specimen (Fig. 4-17a-c). Should tumor tissue be present at this site, differentiation between invasion of the muscle wall and of the prostate can prove difficult.

V

STAGING OF CARCINOMA
OF THE URINARY BLADDER
ON THE BASIS OF MRI RESULTS

5.1 Introduction

This chapter discusses the results obtained with MRI for TNM staging of carcinoma of the urinary bladder (UBC). In order to assess the value of diagnostic investigative techniques, they should be compared with a reference value, which is also referred to in the American literature as the 'golden standard'.[84]

In section 5.2, the histologic findings on cystectomy and autopsy specimens are used as a reference. The staging results from the clinical staging method, CT, MRI, and lymphography are compared with the histologic findings (40 patients). Cystectomy was only indicated in some of the patients with UBC (patients with a tumor staged as T2-T4A N0 M0 with insufficient response to radiotherapy), and autopsy was performed on two cadavers. Hence, on the basis of comparison with histologic findings, a decision could only be reached about the value of MRI in stage T2-T4A N0 M0 tumors.

To evaluate MRI in patients with superficial bladder tumors, who had not undergone cystectomy, it was necessary to choose a different reference. For this group, the clinical staging method was adopted as the reference. In an attempt to increase the reliability of this reference, the outcomes of a 9-month to 3-year follow-up also were included for these patients. This group of patients is discussed in sections 5.3. and 5.4. In section 5.3, the staging results of MRI and CT are compared with the reference (43 patients). In section 5.4, the findings of MRI are compared with those of this reference (51 patients).

As CT is, to date, the most frequently used imaging technique for staging UBC, this chapter pays particular attention to the value of CT relative to that of MRI. As well as determining the accuracy of staging by CT and MRI with respect to the reference values (sections 5.2 and 5.3), a survey is presented of the difference in staging results obtained with these two techniques (section 5.3.2).

5.1.1 Survey of groups of patient

Between January 1986 and August 1988, a total of 172 MRI examinations were performed in 142 patients with a malignant process in the urinary bladder (112 men and 30 women). These were unselected patients of the St. Radboud and Canisius-Wilhelmina Hospital. Because of motion artifacts, the T_2-weighted images could not be assessed in 8 patients (4 at 0.5 T and 4 at 1.5 T) (see also section 3.3.2.2.), so these patients were excluded from this study.

Until January 1987, the MRI study was carried out in Best (Philips Medical Systems Division), where 41 MRI examinations were performed in 37 patients (31 men and 6 women) at a field strength of 0.5 T (Gyroscan S5). In the other 105 patients (81 men and 24 women), 131 MRI examinations were conducted at a field strength of 1.5 T (Gyroscan S15) (University Hospital, Utrecht).

The average age of the patients was 62 years (range, 35-90 years). Table 17 presents a survey of the histologic typing of the tumors. Table 18 looks at the various groups of patients, as discussed in the following sections.

Table 17 **Histological diagnosis of malignant tumors in urinary bladder *).**

	0.5 T	1.5 T	total group
Urothelial cell ca.	24	93	117
Urothelial cell + adeno ca.	1	1	2
Urothelial cell + squamous cell ca.	0	2	2
Squamous cell ca.	1	3	4
Anaplastic ca.	5	1	6
Mesonephrogenic malignant tumor	1	0	1
Leiomyosarcoma	1	0	1
Endometrial ca. in the bladder wall	0	1	1
Total number of patients	33	101	134

*) Excluding 8 patients in whom the T_2 weighted images could not be assessed.

5.2 Evaluation of MRI, CT and the clinical staging method compared with postoperative histopathologic staging based on cystectomy or autopsy specimens

5.2.1 Patients and methods

Within the framework of staging a histologically proved bladder carcinoma, the following examinations were performed in 40 patients (30 men and 10 women; average age, 65 years; age range, 41-78 years):
- clinical staging method according to UICC[215] (see section 1.2.2 (in 40 patients),
- MRI (in 40 patients),
- CT scan (in 37 patients), and
- lymphography (in 23 patients).

This study considered only the results of MRI and CT examinations immediately preceding cystectomy.

CT

CT was performed with third generation CT scanners (Siemens Somatom DR3 and Philips Tomoscan 350). Images were made at a slice thickness of 8 mm, from the diaphragm to the pubic symphysis. A scan interval of 8 mm was maintained in the upper abdomen; the pelvic sections were contiguous.

The CT assessment was performed as described by Hodson et al.;[105] the tumors were grouped according to the TNM stages.[215] It was not possible to distinguish between stages Ta, T1, T2 and T3A on CT, so these stages were grouped together as Ta-T3A. These tumors are characterized by thickening of the bladder wall. Stage T3B indicates a loss of definition of the bladder wall at the transition to perivesical fat or the eruption of a tumor mass into the perivesical fat. In stage T4A, the tumor extends into neighbouring organs. This can be recognized by the disappearance of the fatty tissue normally present between the urinary bladder and these organs. In stage T4B, invasion of the tumor mass is visible in the internal obturator muscle or in the pelvis or abdominal wall.

Lymph nodes were considered abnormal if their diameter exceeded 1.5 cm or if there was clear left-right asymmetry of the iliac nodes.

Table 18 Final tumor staging.

	number of patients (n)		
	MRI + CT + cystectomy (n = 40)	MRI + CT, without cystectomy (n = 43)	MRI, without CT, without cystectomy (n = 51)
	section 5.2	section 5.3	section 5.4
T stages			
T0	8	12	14
Ta-1	3	7	28
T2	2	2	1
T3A	8	15	6
T3B	11	1	0
T4A	2	4	2
T4B	6	2	0
N stages			
N0	32	8	0
N+	8	10	0
Nx	0	25	51
M stages			
M0	36	36	48
M+	4	7	3

MRI

MRI was performed in 11 patients with the Gyroscan S5 at a field strength of 0.5 T and in 29 patients with the Gyroscan S15 at a field strength of 1.5 T. The optimal image was acquired by using a double surface coil at 0.5 T, as described in section 3.4. At a field strength of 1.5 T, a suboptimal double surface coil was used in 9 patients. Images were produced in the transverse, coronal and sagittal planes by using the optimal T_1-weighted sequence described in Chapter 3. Then a series of images was made in at least one plane with a T_2-weighted sequence (also described in Chapter 3).

The slice thickness was 8 mm, with an interval of 1 mm. From the symphysis pubis to the aorta bifurcation, images of the abdomen were acquired at 0.5 T and at 1.5 T as far as the bottom of the kidneys. The patient was prepared as described in section 3.2. The average duration of the MRI examination was 60 min per patient.

Tumor staging was performed with MRI according to the scheme based on the TNM staging system as described by Fisher et al.[76] (see section 3.4.1.1). According to these authors, MRI could not be used to differentiate stages Ta, T1 and T2. These were, therefore, treated as one stage Ta-T2.

Lymphography

On the lymphograms, nodes were considered to be abnormal if they showed a local filling defect and/or enlargement. A final assessment of the MRI examinations was not made until all the MRI examinations, described in this book, had been completed. This assessment was performed independently by two radiologists who had no prior knowledge of the patient's name, the ultimate diagnosis or the outcomes of the other methods of examination. The CT scans and lymphograms were assessed in the same manner. If there was a difference of opinion (14 times in the MR images, 18 times in the CT scans, 5 times in the lymphograms), the final stage was established by mutual consent.

The clinical staging method was performed by the urologist and the pathologist-anatomist, according to UICC guidelines[215] (see section 1.2.2). In 30 patients, the MRI and CT examinations were perfor-

med after the clinical staging method and transurethral resection. In the other 10, clinical staging was done after MRI and CT. A maximum of 5 weeks elapsed between clinical staging and cystectomy, except in 4 patients, in whom the interval was 2½ months. During the intervening period, these 4 patients received radiotherapy or chemotherapy. No treatment was administered to the other patients, between the clinical staging method, the MRI examination, the CT scanning and the cystectomy.

There was never more than a 2-week interval between the CT and MRI examinations. Within 2 weeks of completing the last staging technique, radical cystectomy and pelvic lymphadenectomy (38 patients) or autopsy (2 cadavers) were performed. By means of histologic examination of the cystectomy specimen the histopathologic p.TNM stage was defined.

In order to improve interpretation of the in vivo MR images, in 11 patients, in vitro MR images of the resected specimen were obtained in addition to the in vivo MR images made before cystectomy. The technique has been described in Chapter 4. These images also were assessed according to the TNM staging system.

5.2.2   Results

5.2.2.1   *Patients*

In order to clarify the results, they are split into those for T staging, those for N staging, and those for M staging.

T staging

The results of the clinical staging method, the MRI examination and the CT scanning are presented in Table 19.

Of the eight patients in whom postoperative histopathologic examination revealed no remaining tumor (stage pT0), the clinical staging method had found tumor in six patients (T1 in one patient, T2 in two patients, and T3A in three patients). In four of these patients (stages T2 and T3A), the period between the clinical staging method and the final cystectomy was long (2½ months), owing to administration of chemotherapy or radiotherapy.

In the other two patients (stages T1 and T2), the transurethral resection, which was part of the clinical staging method, was apparently complete. There-

Table 19 A Results of staging by the clinical staging method (T stage).

	cystectomy / autopsy staging							
	pT0	pT1	pT2	pT3A	pT3B	pT4A	pT4B	
clinical staging method								
T0	2	—	—	—	—	—	—	
T1	1	3	—	—	1	—	—	
T2	2	—	2	4	2	—	2	
T3A	3	—	—	4	8	—	2	
T3B	—	—	—	—	0	—	—	
T4A	—	—	—	—	—	2	2	
T4B	—	—	—	—	—	—	0	
n	8	3	2	8	11	2	6	40

Table 19 B Results of staging with MRI (T stage).

	cystectomy / autopsy staging							
	pT0	pT1	pT2	pT3A	pT3B	pT4A	pT4B	
MRI stage								
T0	3	—	—	—	—	—	—	
Ta-2	5	3	2	—	—	—	—	
T3A	—	—	—	5	—	—	—	
T3B	—	—	—	3	10	—	—	
T4A	—	—	—	—	1	2	—	
T4B	—	—	—	—	—	—	6	
n	8	3	2	8	11	2	6	40

Table 19 C Results of staging with CT (T stage).

	cystectomy / autopsy staging							
	pT0	pT1	pT2	pT3A	pT3B	pT4A	pT4B	
CT stage								
T0	1	—	—	—	—	—	—	
Ta-3A	4	2	2	4	—	1	1	
T3B	—	—	—	2	8	—	1	
T4A	2	1	—	1	3	1	—	
T4B	1	—	—	—	—	—	2	
n	8	3	2	7	11	2	4	37

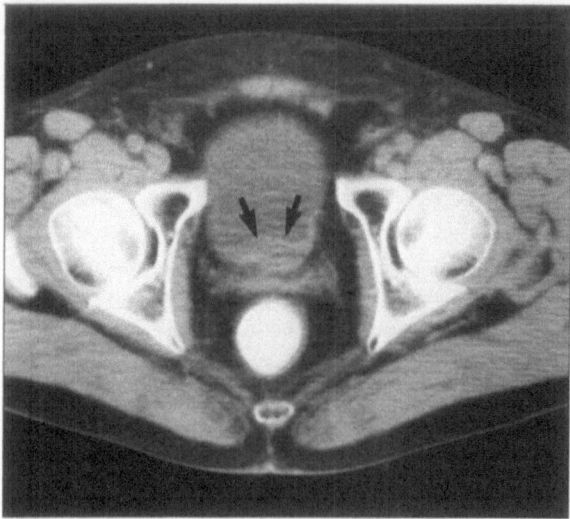 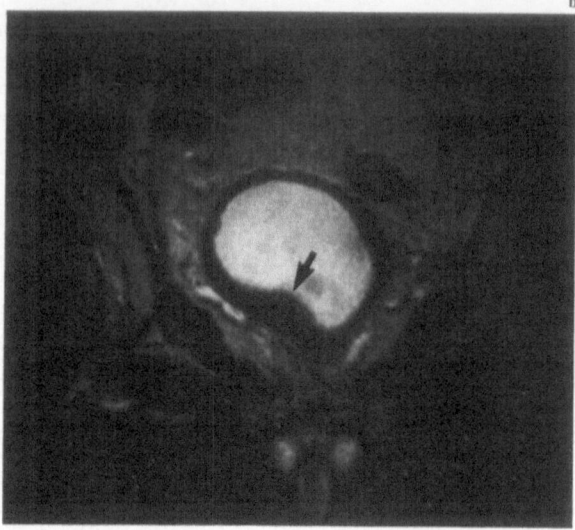

Fig. 5-1. (a) On the CT scan, thickening of the urinary bladder wall can be seen dorsally (arrows), compatible with a stage Ta-T3A tumor. **(b)** On the T2-weighted MR image (1.5 T; SE/2000/100/2), this has just as low a signal intensity as the bladder wall (arrow), indicating fibrosis (stage T0). This was confirmed histologically (see also Fig. 3-5).

fore, the results of the clinical staging method in these six patients cannot be compared with those of the postoperative histopathologic staging.

In the same group of eight patients, in whom the postoperative histopathologic examination did not reveal a tumor, MRI and CT did diagnose a tumor in five and seven patients, respectively. As the clinical staging method preceded the MRI and CT examinations in these patients, this overstaging could have been caused by the inflammatory and granular tissue resulting from the earlier transurethral resection. An example of correct staging by MRI and overstaging

by CT in this group is given in Fig. 5-1. In this patient MRI could indicate, on the basis of T_2-weighted images, that a local thickening of the wall was due to fibrous and granulation tissue, something that was not possible with CT.

In 31 of the 32 patients in whom the postoperative histopathologic examination revealed tumor, the clinical staging method could differentiate correctly between stages pTa-T1 and pT2 or higher.

With MRI, it was possible in all cases to distinguish between stage pTa-pT2 tumors (5 patients) and

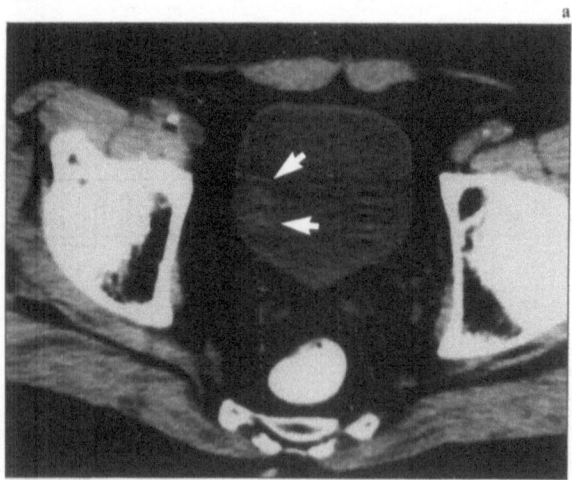 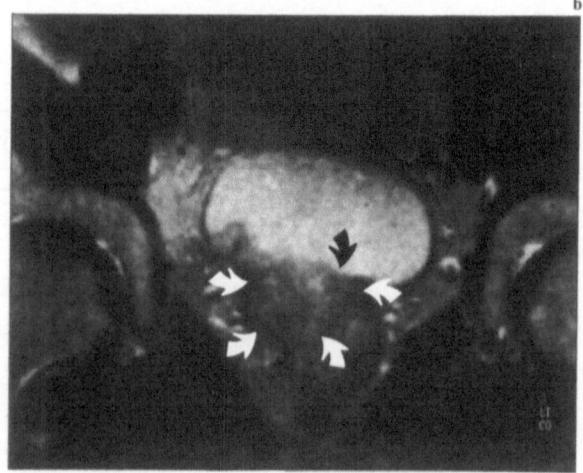

Fig. 5-2. (a) On the CT scan a papillary tumor can be seen (stage Ta-T3A) (arrows). The other CT scans reveal no abnormalities. **(b)** On the coronal T2-weighted MR image (1.5 T; SE/2000/100/2), one can see invasion of the prostate (curved arrows, stage T4A). This was confirmed histologically.

tumors in stage pT3A or higher (27 patients). This differentiation could not be made with CT. The clinical staging method also had trouble with this distinction: in 9 of the 27 patients with a tumor in stage pT3A or higher, this technique staged the tumors as Ta-T2. The difference in staging as Ta-T2 and T3A or higher, by MRI and the clinical staging method is significant (p < .01, McNemar test).

Table 20A-C shows the values of the clinical staging method, MRI and CT for the differentiation of tumors in stages pTa-pT3A and pT3B or higher. It follows from this table that in patients with stage pT3A tumors, MRI and CT overstaged the tumors (in 3 of the 13 and 4 of the 12 patients, respectively). The distinction between stages Ta-T3A and T3B or higher was worst with the clinical staging method, and this

Table 20 A Differentiation between stages ≤ T3A and ≥ T3B by using the clinical staging method.

	cystectomy / autopsy staging		
	pTa-3A	≥ pT3B	number of patients
clinical staging method			
Ta-3A	**13**	15	28
≥ T3B	—	**4 (2*)**	4
n	13	19	32

* number of correct stagings as T3B, T4A and T4B.

Table 20 B Differentiation besteen stages ≤ T3A and ≥ T3B using MRI.

	cystectomy / autopsy staging		
	pTa-3A	≥ pT3B	number of patients
MRI stage			
Ta-3A	**10**	0	10
≥ T3B	3	**19 (18*)**	22
n	13	19	32

* number of correct stagings as T3B, T4A and T4B.

Table 20 C Differentiation between stages ≤ T3A and ≥ T3B using CT.

	cystectomy / autopsy staging		
	pTa-3A	≥ pT3B	number of patients
CT stage			
Ta-3A	**8**	2	10
≥ T3B	4	**15 (11*)**	19
n	12	17	29

* number of correct stagings as T3B, T4A and T4B.

method definitely understaged tumors: in 15 of the 32 patients. The difference in staging as Ta-T3A and T3B or higher by MRI and by the clinical staging method is significant (p < .01, McNemar tests).

With MRI, a correct differentiation between stages pT3B, pT4A, and pT4B was obtained in 18 of the 19 patients with tumors in stages pT3B or higher. This was the case in 2 of the 19 patients when the clinical staging method was used, and in 11 of the 17 patients when CT was used. These differences in staging are significant (p < .01 and p = .03, respectively, McNemar test). Furthermore, the degree of overstaging with CT was much larger in all groups than with MRI. Examples of overstaging with CT and MRI are presented in section 5.2.2.2. An example of understaging with CT is illustrated by Fig. 5-2.

N staging

Table 21A-C presents the staging results of MRI, CT scanning and lymphography for the N stages. Lymphography was not performed in 17 patients. The

Table 21 A   Results of staging with MRI (N stages).

	cystectomy / autopsy staging		
	N0	N+	number of patients
MRI stage			
N0	32	3	35
N+	0	5	5
n	32	8	40

Table 21 B   Results of staging with CT (N stages).

	cystectomy / autopsy staging		
	N0	N+	number of patients
CT stage			
N0	27	4	31
N+	3	3	6
n	30	7	37

Table 21 C   Results of staging with lymphography (N stages).

	cystectomy / autopsy staging		
	N0	N+	number of patients
lymphography stage			
N0	15	4	19
N+	2	2	4
n	17	6	23

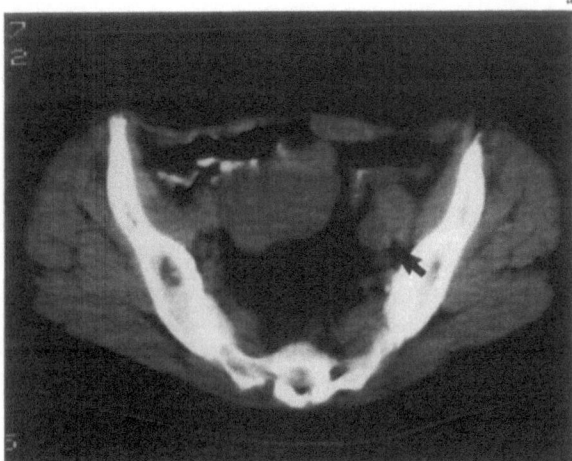
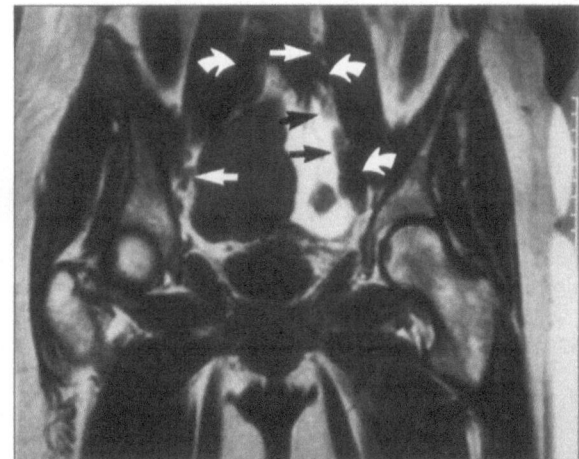

Fig. 5-3. (a) On the CT scan, pathologically enlarged nodes are visible in the left iliac region (arrow). **(b)** On the coronal MR image (1.5 T; SE/750/30/2), however, these appear to be vessels (curved arrows) and normal nodes (arrows). This was confirmed during surgery.

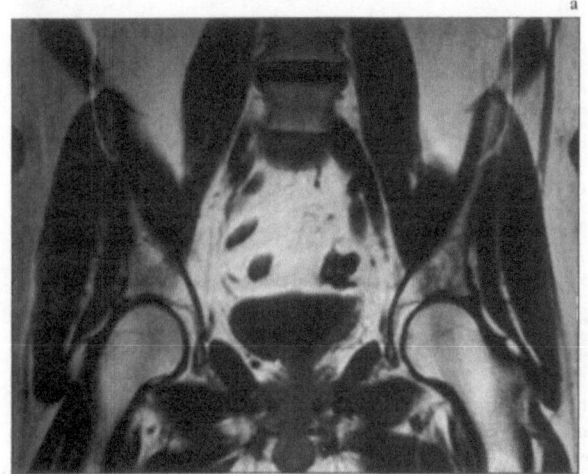
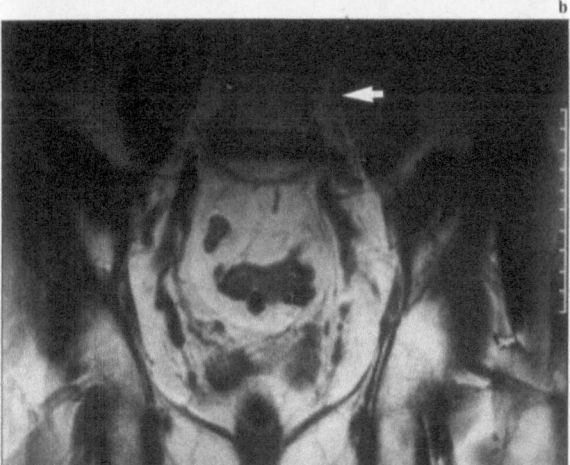

selection of these patients was purely random. MRI showed the highest sensitivity and specificity for N staging (63% and 100%, respectively); it was followed by CT scanning (43% and 90%, respectively) and then lymphography (33% and 88%, respectively). Because of the small number of patients, these differences are not statistically significant.

In three patients the lymph node metastases could not be recognized on MRI, CT or lymphography. These were microscopic metastases in nonenlarged lymph nodes. CT gave an incorrect result in four other patients. The diagnosis was false positive in three cases and false negative in one case (Figs. 5-3

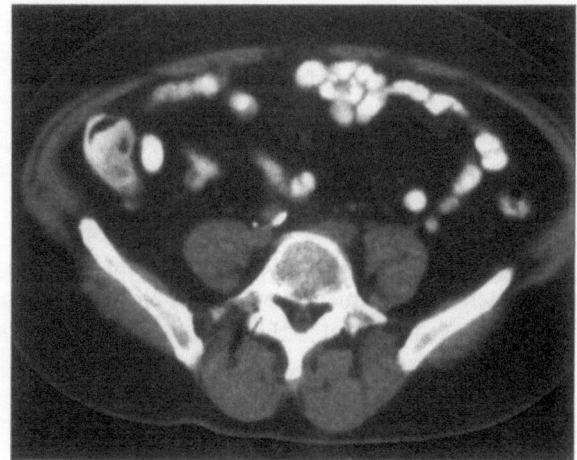

Fig. 5-4. (a) and **(b)** Coronal MR images (1.5 T; SE/800/30/2) made at an interval of 1 year. The MR images demonstrate the growth of a high-iliac node (arrow). Although its size is not abnormal, it is suspected to be a metastasis. **(c)** On the CT-scan, no lymph nodes can be distinguished. During surgery, a lymph node metastasis was found in the left iliacal region.

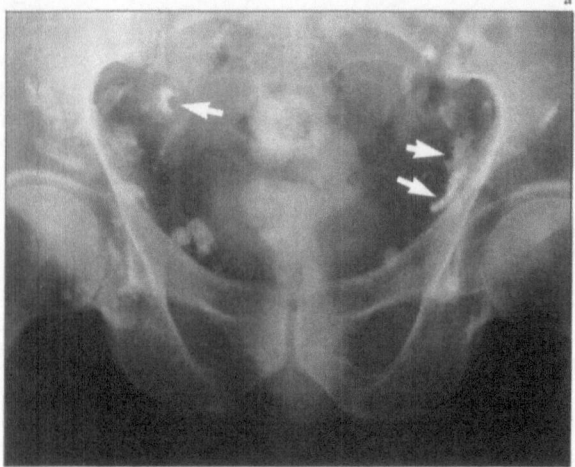
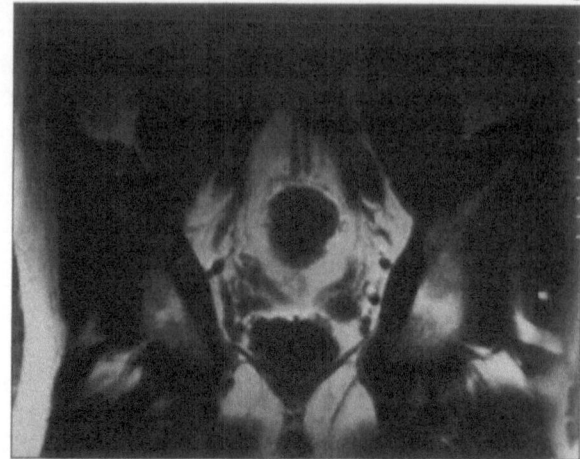

Fig. 5-5. (a) The lymphogram shows iliac, abnormally enlarged nodes with accumulation defects on both sides, compatible with lymph node metastases (arrows). **(b)** On the coronal MR image (1.5 T; SE/800/30/2), however, no abnormally enlarged lymph nodes can be recognized. This was confirmed during surgery.

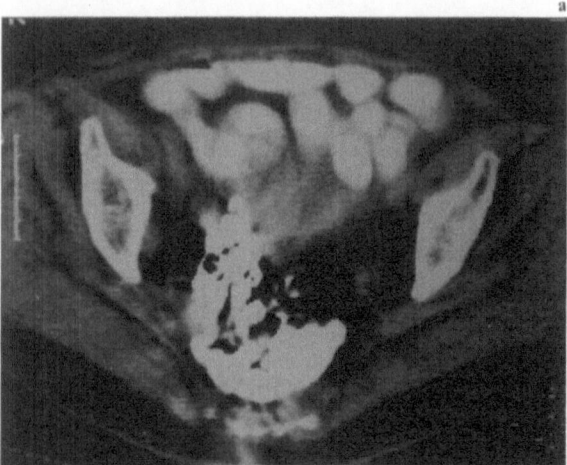
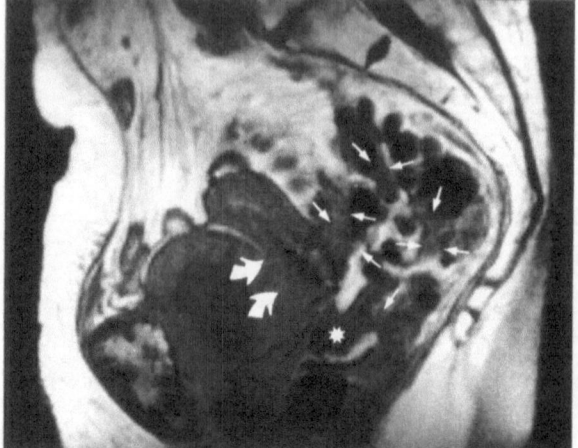

Fig. 5-6. (a) On the CT scan, one can see interference by barium artifacts, but no indications of intraperitoneal metastases. **(b)** On the sagittal MR image (1.5 T; SE/750/30/2), tumor spread can be seen in the cervix and vagina (curved arrows). There are also indications of intraperitoneal metastases (peritonitis carcinomatosa) (arrows) and fluid in the Douglas cul-de-sac (*).

and 5- 4). In three other patients, lymphography gave an incorrect staging: two false-positive and one false-negative diagnosis (Fig. 5-5).

M staging

As MRI was only used to display pelvic structures (0.5 T) and abdominal structures up to the level of the bottom of the kidneys (1.5 T), the determination of the M stage is limited to this area. With regard to the value of MRI compared with that of other diagnostic techniques for tasks such as visualizing liver and lung metastases, no information could be obtained for this very reason.

In 4 of the 40 patients, distant metastases were found

in the region displayed. In 3 patients, this was peritonitis carcinomatosa, while in another, a secondary tumor was found in the sigmoid colon. In 2 of these patients the distant metastases could be recognized on the MR images, but CT did not show them (Fig. 3-22 and 5-6).

5.2.2.2 MR images of resected specimens

No difference was seen in the T staging results of the in vitro and the in vivo MR images. In 3 of the 11 in vitro MR images, identical overstaging was found.

In 1 of the 3 patients, tumor invasion of the vaginal wall (stage T4A) was seen on both in vivo and in vitro MR images and on CT scans. Histologic examina-

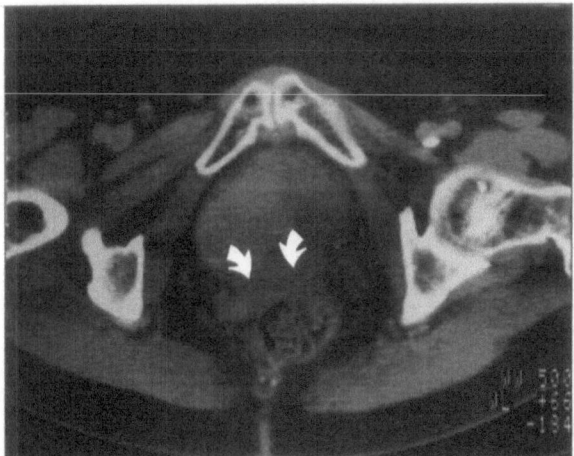

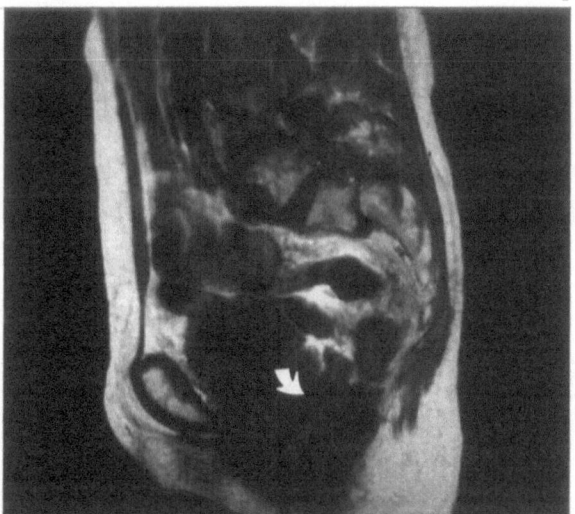

Fig. 5-7. Patient with urothelial cell carcinoma of the entire urinary bladder floor. Both on the CT scan (a), and on the sagittal in vitro (b) and in vivo MR images (c) (1.5 T; SE/750/30/2), the fat layer between bladder tumor and cervix is interrupted, arguing in favor of tumor invasion of the cervix (stage T4A) (curved arrows). Histologic examination of the resected specimen, however, only demonstrated invasion of the perivesical fat (stage T3B).

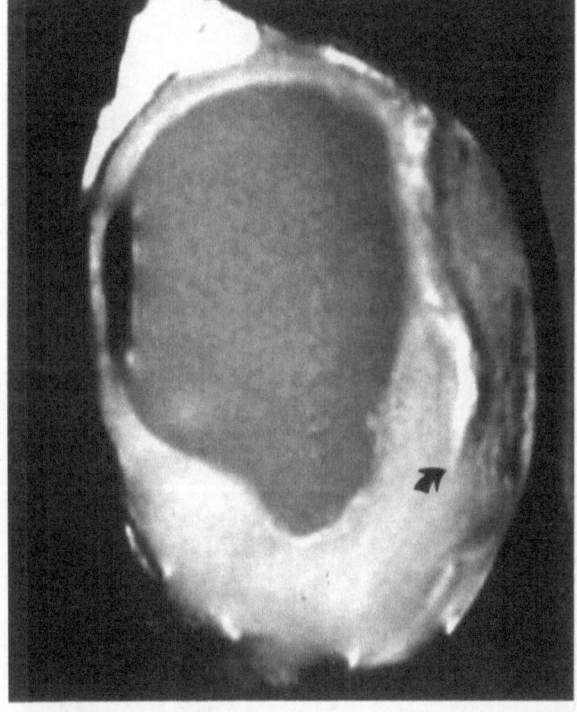

Histologic examination in this patient, however, revealed an exophytic, expansively growing squamous cell carcinoma, without invasion of the perivesical fat (stage T3A). This could be explained by the fact that the manner of growth pattern of this tumor was expansive rather than infiltrative.

tion however, revealed only invasion of the bladder wall (stage T3A) and of the perivesical fat (=stage T3B) (Fig. 5-7). The explanation of the false-positive staging was that the thin fat layer, normally present between bladder wall and vaginal mucous membrane, was missing. As a rule, this layer marks the border between bladder wall and vagina on MR images and CT scans.

In a second patient, tumor invasion of the perivesical fat (stage T3B) could be seen on both the in vivo and in vitro MR images and on CT scans. It also seemed to be present on the macroscopic specimen (Fig. 5-8).

Finally, invasion of the perivesical fat (stage T3B) was visible in the third patient both on MR images before cystectomy, and on the MR images of the resected specimen (Fig. 5-9). The CT scans, however, showed a tumor that was limited to the bladder wall (stage T3A). This was confirmed by histologic examination: evidence was seen of tumor invasion up to but not into the perivesical fat. Furthermore, inflammatory and granulation tissue was present in the perivesical fat, caused by chronic cystitis as a result of self-catheterization. This provided the explanation for the apparent infiltration into the perivesical fat seen on the MR images.

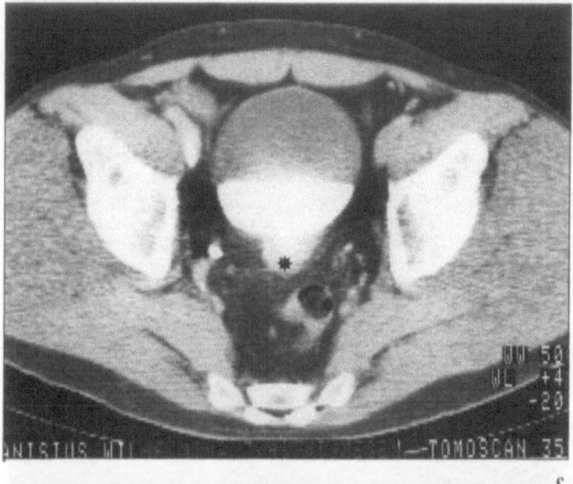

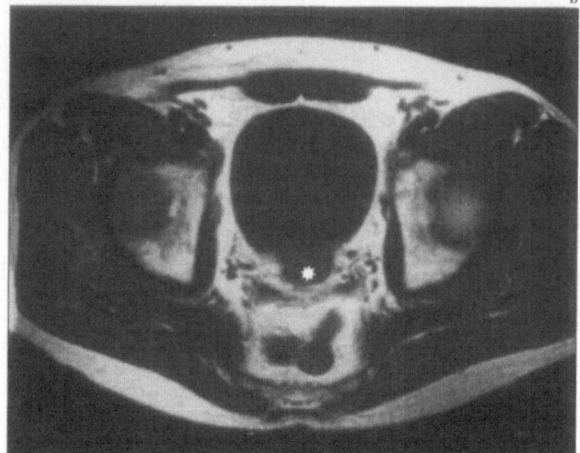

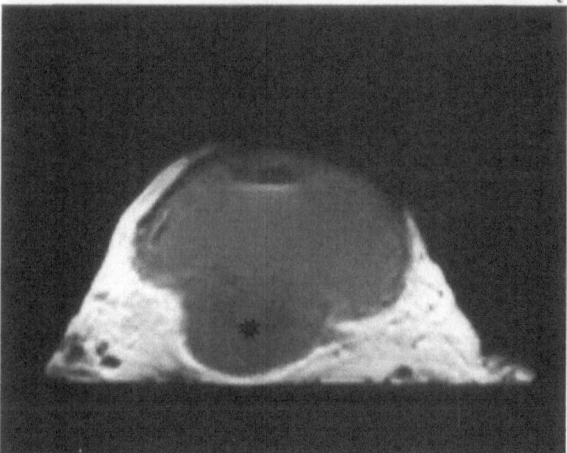

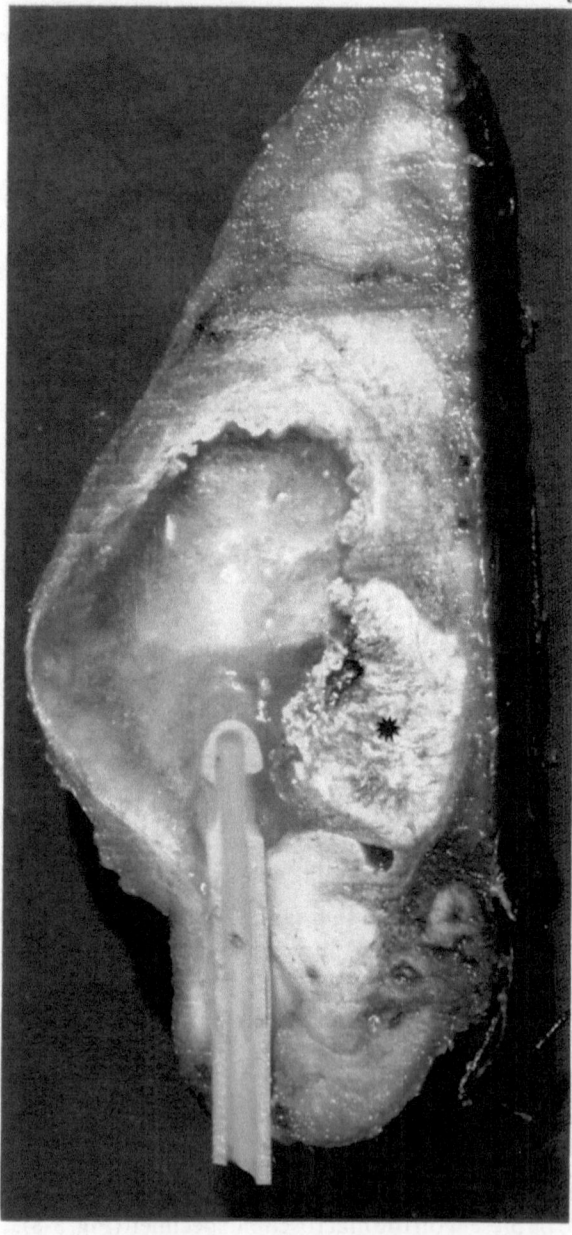

Fig. 5-8. Patient with squamous cell carcinoma (*) at the dorsal wall of the urinary bladder. (a) The CT-scan, and (b) the in vivo and (c) the in vitro MRI images (1.5 T;SE/750/30/2) reveal indications of invasion of the perivesical fat (stage T3B). (d) This also appears to be the case with the resected specimen. Histologic examination, however, revealed an extensively growing tumor, without invasion of the fat (stage T3A).

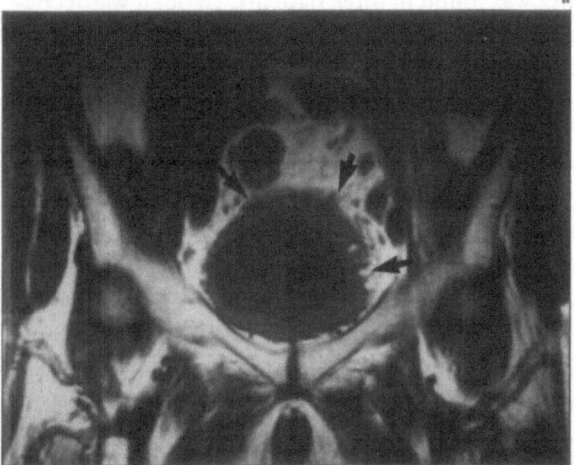
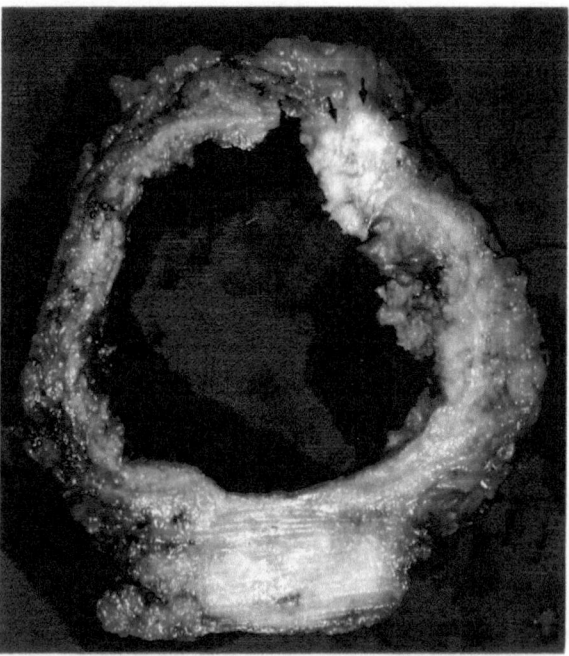

Fig. 5-9. Patient with squamous cell carcinoma of the urinary bladder and chronic cystitis as a result of long-term selfcatheterisation. (a) The coronal MR image (1.5 T, SE/800/30/2) reveals a thickened bladder wall that is not clearly distinguished where it apposes the perivesical fat. This argues in favor of tumor invasion into this fat (stage T3B, arrows). (b) This also appears to be the case at one spot on the resected specimen (arrows). Histologic examination did not, however, reveal any indications of growth into the perivesical fat (stage T3A).

5.2.3. Discussion

T staging

Various reports on the relative values of MRI and CT in staging UBC have been published (Table 7). However, the numbers of patients were not very large in the studies that used postoperative histopathologic staging of cystectomy or autopsy specimens as the reference. The largest series (40 patients) was recently described by Buy et al.[43] and included the same number of patients as in this study. No reports have been published that compare the value of clinical staging with that of staging by use of MRI and CT.

With MRI and CT, it was difficult to differentiate between *residual tumor and infected tissue*. Transurethral resection preceded the MRI or CT study in 30 patients and resulted in overstaging in 5 and 7 patients resp. This problem has also been emphasized by other authors.[76,131] It did appear that with MRI, as already seen in section 3.3.2, one could distinguish between fibrosis and granulation tissue.

With the clinical staging method, staging of tumors in *stages T2 or less* was highly accurate. It should be pointed out, however, that the number of patients

with tumors in these stages was small (n = 13). These findings agree with those of other authors.[14, 115, 135, 164, 223, 228] The staging accuracy of MRI and CT for tumors in these stages cannot be compared with that of the clinical staging method, because differentiation between stages Ta, T1, and T2 is impossible with these imaging techniques.

Differentiation between tumors in *stages T2 or less and T3A or more* by using the clinical staging method proved problematic: it could not be done in 9 of 27 patients. In accordance with the experience of other authors,[13, 43, 76, 188] this *was* possible with MRI. This is all the more important because the distinction cannot be achieved with CT (Table 4).

The staging accuracy of MRI for tumors in *stages T3A or higher* was significantly higher than that of the clinical staging method (p < .01, McNemar test). Other authors also found a low degree of accuracy for clinical staging of tumors in these stages.[152, 202] The reason for this low accuracy is that it is impossible to remove a tumor as far as the exterior of the bladder wall by transurethral resection. One exception is tumor invasion of the prostate (stage T4A).

The only possible way of differentiating tumors of stage T3A or higher is to use the findings of bimanual examination. But this examination is strongly investigator dependent. Furthermore, its value is limited in dorsal tumors, high up in the bladder.

The benefit of MRI over CT was not significant for the differentiation of stage Ta-T3A tumors from tumors in stage T3B or higher. However, the distinction between *stages T3B, T4A and T4B* was significantly better on MRI (p = 0.03, McNemar test).

N staging

Lymph node metastases are important for determining therapeutic policy. Should metastases be present in the iliac or paraaortic lymph nodes, the patient will not be considered for a curative form of therapy. The accuracy of detection of these nodes was higher with MRI than with CT. Published results of MRI and CT are equal (Tables 6 and 7, sections 1.3.3 and 1.3.5). The better staging results obtained with MRI in this study may be explained by the fact that images in three directions were used for the determination of lymph node metastases, whereas in the literature, only images in the transverse plane were used. An important point is that MRI did not show any false-positive diagnoses. A false-positive diagnosis was established in three patients with CT: vessels and intestine were mistaken for abnormally enlarged lymph nodes.

MRI also appears to produce better staging results than does lymphography; yet on the basis of published data, one might well expect that lymphography would be better able to display the small cores in lymph nodes.[59, 130, 138, 177, 212] A possible reason is the inability of lymphography to display nodes along the internal iliac artery, something that MRI can do. The accuracy of lymphography in this patient group was slightly lower than that reported in the literature (see Table 6, section 1.3.4). The number of patients in whom both lymphography and MRI were performed was relatively small (23 patients). The number of patients with lymph node metastases in this group was even smaller (6 patients). We, therefore, must be careful in drawing any definite conclusions. This will be discussed further in section 5.3.

M staging

This study has addressed itself primarily to the gene-

ration of images of pelvic structures. With regard to the presence of distant metastases, only pelvic metastases were considered, for example, metastases in neighbouring organs, peritonitis carcinomatosa, or bone marrow metastases. Peritonitis carcinomatosa was found in three patients. In on, it was recognized only on the MR images. In another patient, a metastasis was found in the sigmoid colon. This too could be recognized only on MRI.

5.2.4 Interim conclusions

The clinical staging method appears to be very reliable in differentiating between *infection and tumor tissue* and in staging tumors in *stages Ta, T1, and T2*. In these patients, both MRI and CT have their limitations. Conversely, MRI is more accurate in staging tumors in *stages T3A, T3B, T4A and T4B*; it is precisely in this range that clinical staging and staging by CT fail.

In 23 patients who also underwent lymphography, MRI appears to be more accurate than lymphography and CT in detecting lymph node metastases.

In the group of patients discussed here, histologic examination of the resected specimen was chosen as the reference value. This does, however, imply a certain selection: only urothelial cell carcinomas staged as T2-T4A N0 M0 that do not react sufficiently to radiotherapy or that occur together with carcinoma in situ, and nonurothelial cell carcinomas in the same stages are considered for cystectomy. Hence, the number of patients with tumors staged as Ta-T2 and the number with lymph node metastases and distant metastases was small. One must, therefore, be cautious about generalizing from these data.

5.3 Evaluation of staging with MRI and CT by using a combination of clinical staging and follow-up as a reference

In order to obtain an overall impression of the staging value of MRI in *all* tumor stages, one also must evaluate the patients who did not undergo cystectomy.

These included:
a. patients with urothelial cell carcinoma with a low degree of malignancy (G1-2) staged as Ta N0 M0 and T1 N0 M0,

b. patients with urothelial cell carcinoma with a higher degree of malignancy (G3) and/or staged as T2 N0 M0, T3A N0 M0, or T3B N0 M0, who no longer had any vital tumor tissue in the urinary bladder after radiotherapy (40 Gy),

c. patients with tumors in stages T4 N0 M0, and

d. patients with metastases in lymph nodes or with distant metastases (N+ or M+).

In these patients, the histopathologic data on the resected specimen were not available; therefore, results of clinical staging method were used as reference values. In order to increase the reliability of this reference value, the outcomes of a follow-up of 9 months to 3 years also were included for this group. These patients could be split into one group who underwent MRI and CT and one group in whom only MRI was performed. The first group will be discussed in this section, the other in section 5.4.

To obtain an optimal evaluation of MRI compared with CT for T staging, the results of CT and MRI for all patients who underwent these examinations (i.e., including the patients from section 5.2) are presented in section 5.3.2.

5.3.1 Patients and method

Within the framework of the staging sytem a histologically proved UBC, the following examinations were performed out in 43 patients (35 men and 8 women):

- clinical staging by the UICC method (43 patients),
- MRI (43 patients)
- CT (43 patients), and
- lymphography (22 patients).

Table 22 A Results of staging with MRI (T stages).

	clinical staging method (incl. follow-up)			
	T0	Ta-1	≥ T2	number of patients
MRI stage				
T0	7	1	—	
Ta-2	3	5	1 (1)	
≥ T3A	2 (2)	1 (1)	23 (15)	
	12	7	23	43

( ) = patients in whom recurrence of tumor was found during follow-up.

Table 22 B Results of staging with CT (T stages).

	clinical staging method (incl. follow-up)			
	T0	Ta-1	≥ T2	number of patients
CT stage				
T0	3	3	2	
Ta-3A	4	3	7 (4)	
≥ T3B	5 (2)	1 (1)	15 (10)	
	12	7	24	43

( ) = patients in whom recurrence of tumor was found during follow-up.

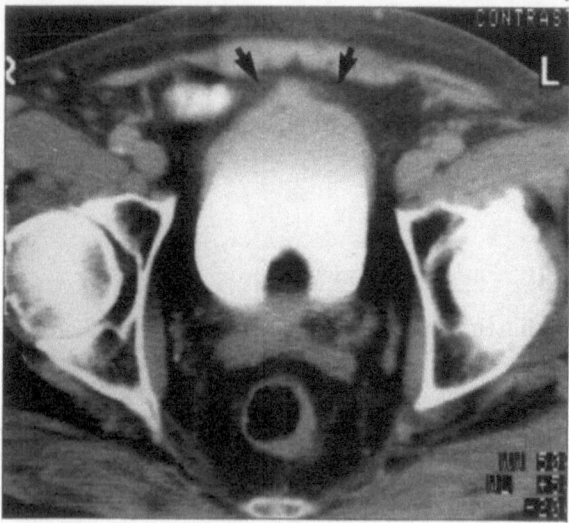
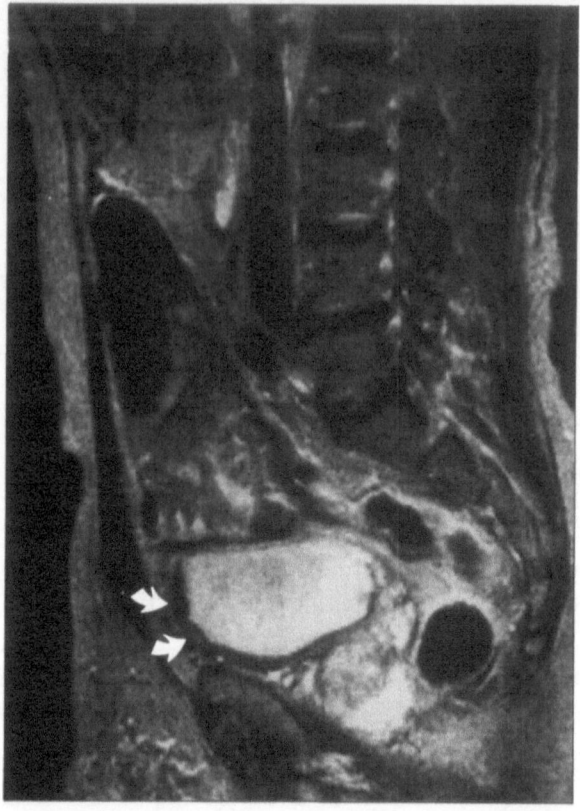

Fig. 5-10. (a) On the CT scan, one can see a ventral thickening of the urinary bladder wall with a lack of definition in the perivesical fat (arrows, stage T3B). **(b)** The sagittal T2-weighted MR image (1.5 T; SE/2000/100/2) reveals an abnormally high signal intensity at the thickened wall (curved arrows), compatible with a malignant tumor infiltrating the deeper muscle layer (stage T3A) (see also Fig. 3-7). The clinical staging method, however, revealed only infection and granulation tissue (stage T0).

This study only considered those patients in whom clinical staging was performed within 4 weeks of the MRI and CT examinations. This was followed by accurate follow-up, consisting of urethrocystoscopy and cytologic urinanalysis every 3 months during the first year, and thereafter, less frequently (every 4/5/6 months). If relapse was suspected macroscopically, differentiated transurethral resection was performed, followed by histologic study.

In those patients in whom a lymphography had been performed check-up images of the lymph nodes were made after 6 weeks, 3 months, and then biannually. The period between the CT and MRI examinations did not exceed 3 weeks. The technique and assessment criteria of CT scanning and MRI were in accordance with those described in section 5.2. It was not possible to have the MR images and CT scans from this group of patients evaluated separately by two radiologists, so they were assessed only by the first author.

5.3.2   Results

T staging

In 29 patients, before MRI, CT, and clinical staging,

a transurethral resection was performed. The gap between this previous resection and the other studies was at least 3 months. In these patients, tumor relapse of a UBC treated much earlier by transurethral resection was suspected.

The follow-up period was 9 to 36 months (average, 18 months). The results of the MRI and CT studies are presented in Tables 22A and 22B. Because published data[152, 202] and our own results (section 5.2) seem to indicate that clinical staging is not reliable for tumors in stages T2 or higher (except for tumor invasion of the prostate), these stages have been combined. In this table, the number of patients who suffered a relapse during the follow-up period is given in parentheses.

In 6 of the 19 patients *with no malignant neoplasm* or with a *stage Ta or T1 tumor*, MRI resulted in overstaging. Understaging was seen in one patient in this group. With CT, tumors in 10 patients were found to be overstaged and 3 were understaged. The overstaging with CT was quite considerable in 6 patients: a stage T0 or Ta-T1 tumor was mistaken on the CT scan for a malignant tumor (stage T3B or higher) that had minimally infiltrated the perivesical fat (Fig. 5-10).

In 3 patients, there was tumor relapse within 3 to 6 months after clinical staging. One of the patients died as a result of this. In these patients both MRI and CT overstaged the tumors. In all patients in whom there was overstaging by either MRI or CT, a transurethral resection had been performed earlier.

Of the 24 patients in whom the tumor was staged as *T2 or higher* by the clinical staging, 16 later had tumor relapse. As a result, eight of them died. Eight patients remained free of tumor (after 66 Gy radiotherapy). In these 24 patients, the tumor was staged with MRI as Ta-T2 in 1 patient and T3A or higher in 23 patients. CT failed to detect a tumor of stage T2 or higher in 2 patients, whereas MRI actually staged the tumor correctly (Fig. 5-11).

In 4 patients, histologic evidence was seen of tumor invasion of the *prostate*. This could be seen on the MR images of all patients, something that could not be achieved with CT in 3 patients. The CT staging of tumors in these 3 patients was T0, T3B and T4B.

Table 23 presents a survey of the staging results of MRI and CT including patients from section 5.2. It can be seen from this table that the percentage agreement is small (50%, standard deviation 3%). Furthermore, there was no shift to any particular side. From this, one can conclude that these two techniques produced significantly different staging results. The largest difference was seen in stage T0 (agreement between MRI and CT in 18% of the patients). The smallest difference was found in stage T3B (agreement in 71% of the patients).

N staging

In the group of 43 patients, 22 lymphographic examinations were performed, 4 of which could not be included in this study because of technical problems (insufficient contrast in the lymphatic system and/or too small a field of view with the 0.5 T sandwich coil).

In Table 24, the results of MRI and CT are compared with those of lymphography backed up by follow-up. On the lymphograms, there was no doubt about the presence or absence of lymph node metastases. Ten patients had obviously pathologically enlarged lymph nodes with filling defects. In the other 8, the lymphogram was completely normal. In these 18 patients, the follow-up period was 1-3 years (average, 2 years).

The images of node metastases on the lymphograms in 2 of the 10 patients were confirmed by needle biopsy. The suspicion of lymph node metastases in the other 8 patients was reinforced by the clinical course: 6 died as a result of tumor; there was a simultaneous increase in the filling defects in the lymph nodes and in the UBC. In the other 2 patients, after chemotherapy or radiotherapy there was a synchronous decrease in the bladder tumor and of the filling defects in the lymph nodes.

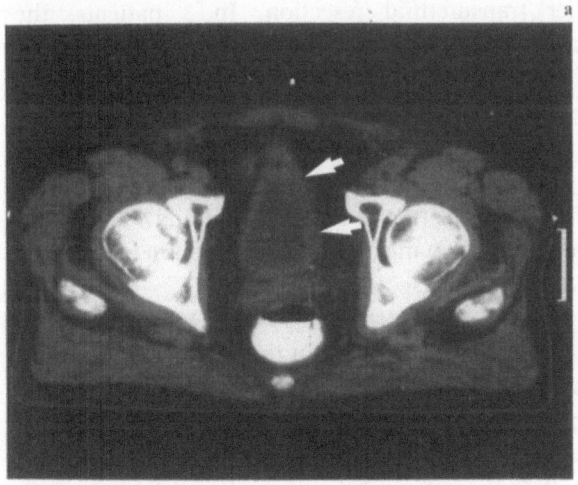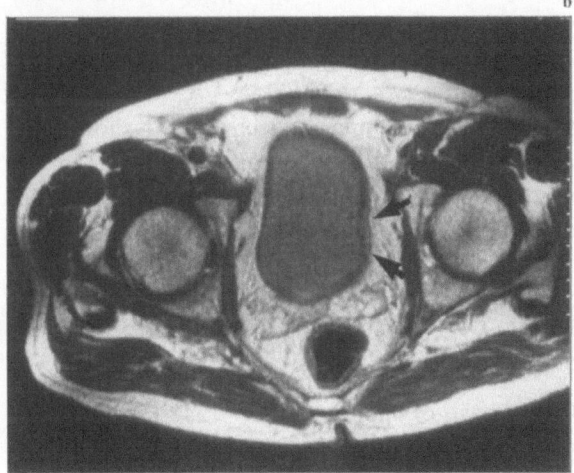

Fig. 5-11. (a) The CT scan shows a slight thickening of the wall, compatible with local hypertrophy (stage T0) (arrows). **(b)** The transverse MR image (0.5 T; SE/2000/60/2) reveals a raised signal intensity at the wall thickening, in keeping with a tumor (stage T3A) (arrows). This was confirmed by the clinical staging method.

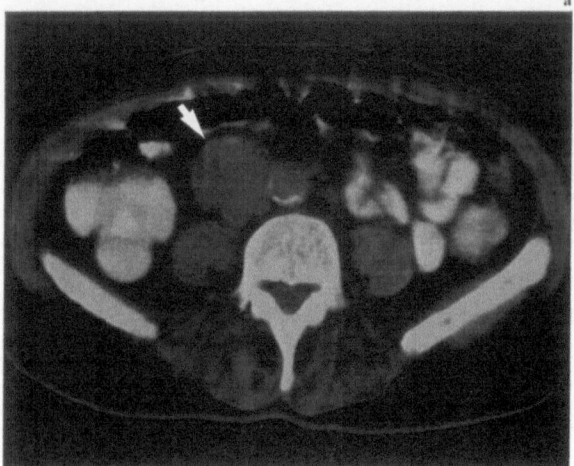 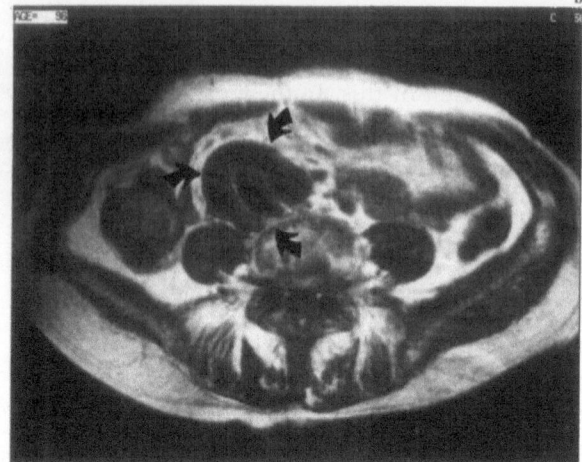

Fig. 5-12. (a) The CT scan shows something that could be lymph node metastases (arrow). **(b)** Thanks to the flow-void phenomenon, the transverse MR image (1.5 T; SE/750/30/2) shows that these are very elongated vessels (arrows).

The 8 patients with normal lymphograms showed no change during the follow-up period.

All lymph node metastases were detected with MRI, without false-positive results. CT failed to find the metastases in one patient, and in two others, vessels were mistaken for pathologic lymphomas (Fig. 5-12).

M staging

With MRI, bone marrow metastases were shown in the pelvis or the lumbar vertebral column in 7 of the 43 patients. In 2, this finding was proved by biopsy. In the other 5, the suspicion was supported by follow-up. In all these patients, conventional radiography and CT were performed, and in 4 bone scintigraphy also was performed. Conventional radiography was positive in 1 of the 7 patients, in 2 the CT was positive, and skeletal scintigraphy was positive in 2 of the 4 patients (Fig. 5-13).

MRI was the only imaging technique to show bone marrow metastases in 2 patients (Fig. 5-14). In the other 36, the clinical course did not give any indication of bone marrow metastases.

5.3.3   Discussion

T staging

On the basis of published data[14, 115, 135, 164, 218, 223, 228] and our own results (see section 5.2), the accuracy of clinical staging for tumors in stages lower than T2 seems to be high. The group of patients described in this section consists of 19 patients in whom the

tumor was clinically staged as lower than T2. In 16 of these patients, no relapse was seen during the follow-up period. This supports the hypothesis that the tumor was completely removed during clinical staging. Considering these and published results, the clinical staging method in these 16 patients is a reliable reference. The 3 patients in whom a relapse occurred will be discussed later.

Of the 16 patients with tumors staged as T0, Ta, or T1 who showed no relapse, MRI overstaged the tumor in 3 and understaged in one. With CT, the results were clearly worse: overstaging in 7 patients, understaging in 3 patients. The reason for the overstaging with both techniques was the inability to distinguish tumor from infected tissue caused by an earlier transurethral resection. In 3 patients, the overstaging produced by CT was qualitatively very large (T3B, T4A, and T4B). These patients were not going to be considered for curative therapy on the basis of the CT results. The difference in staging is explained by the inability of CT to differentiate fibrous from tumor tissue. According to Ebner et al.,[62] MRI can make this differentiation in a case of 'late' fibrosis (see also Chapter 3).

In three patients in whom the tumor was clinically staged as stage T0 (two patients) or Ta-T1 (one patient), a tumor relapse occurred within 6 months of this staging and an invasive tumor was established. In these three patients, staging with MRI was as follows: T3A (once) and T3B (twice), and with CT: T3B (three times). One wonders whether the tumor

Table 23   Results of staging with MRI versus CT (T stages).

	MRI stage					
	T0	Ta-3A	T3B	T4A	T4B	
CT stage						
T0	**2**	7	—	1	—	
Ta-3A	5	**17**	3	1	1	
T3B	1	5	**12**	2	1	
T4A	2	5	2	**4**	1	
T4B	1	1	—	1	**5**	
n	11	35	17	9	8	80
% agreement between MRI and CT	18	49	71	44	63	50

Table 24 A   Results of staging with MRI (N stages).

	lymphography staging (incl. follow-up)		
	N0	N+	number of patients
MRI stage			
N0	**8**	0	**8**
N+	0	**10**	**10**
n	**8**	**10**	**18**

Table 24 B   Results of staging with CT (N stages).

	lymphography staging (incl. follow-up)		
	N0	N+	number of patients
CT stage			
N0	**6**	1	**7**
N+	2	**9**	**11**
n	**8**	**10**	**18**

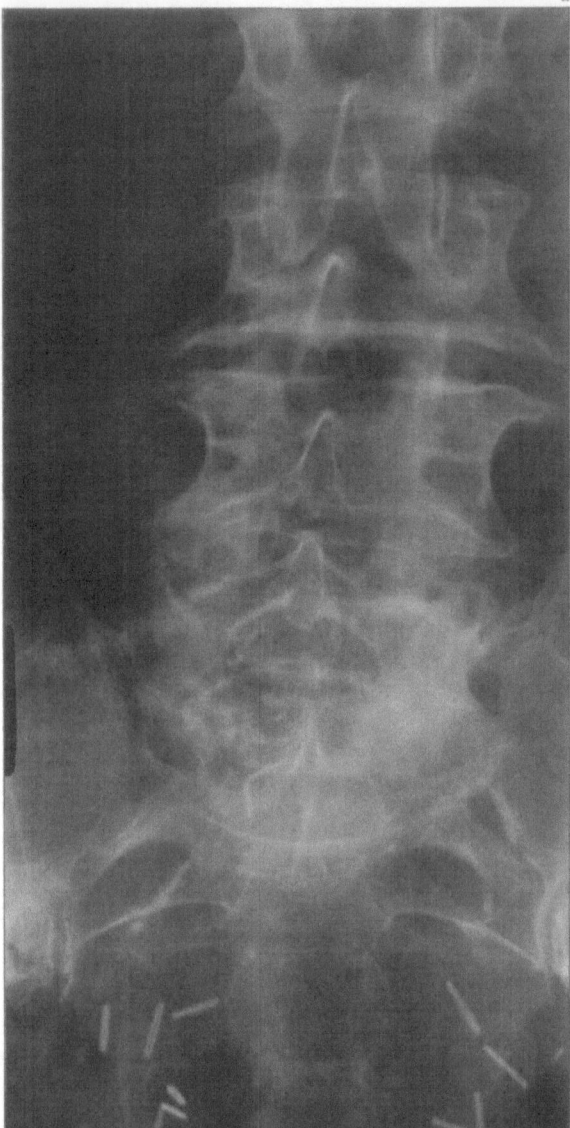

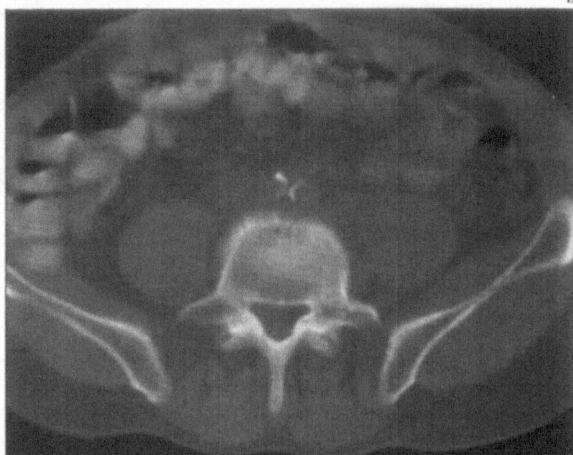

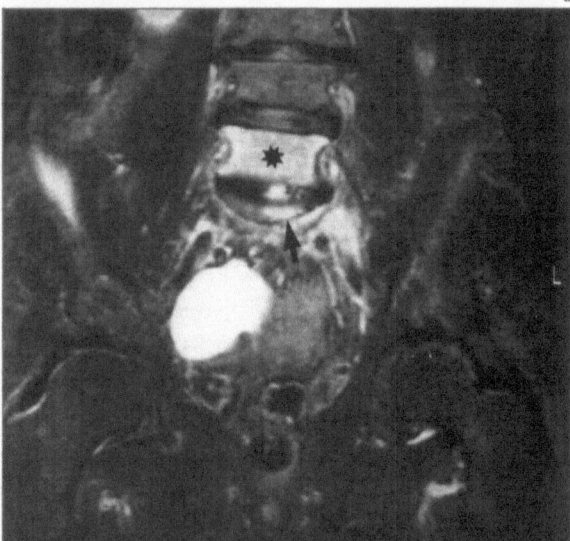

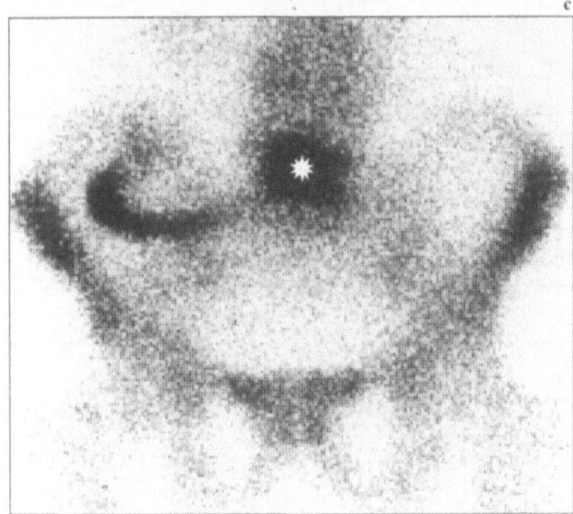

Fig. 5-13. (a) Conventional radiograph of the lumbar vertebral column and **(b)** CT scan show that the bone structure of L4 is normal. **(c)** Both the skeletal scintigram and **(d)** the coronal MR image (1.5 T; IR/2000/100/30/2), however, reveal indications of bone marrow metastases in this vertebral body (*). The MR image also shows a metastasis in the body of L5 (arrow).

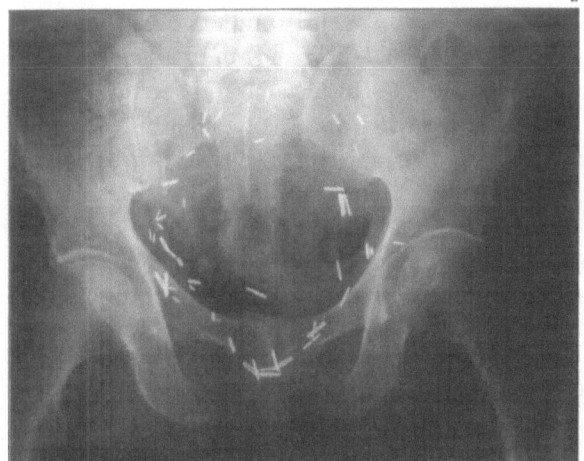

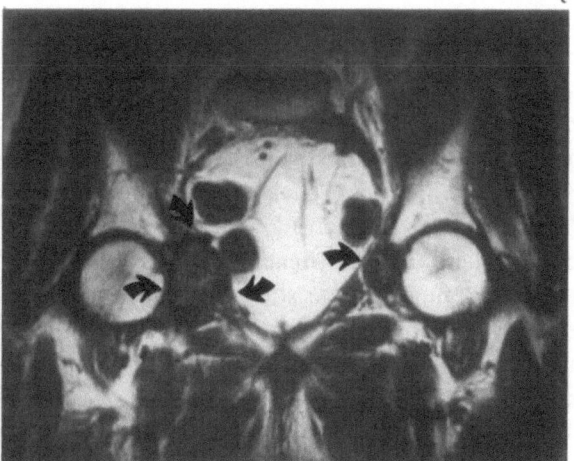

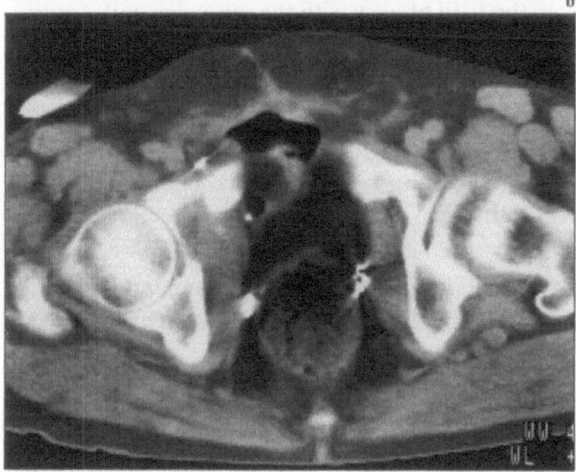

Fig. 5-14. (a) Conventional radiograph and **(b)** CT scan with no abnormalities. **(c)** On the MR image (1.5 T; SE/800/30/2), a diseased region can be seen bilaterally at the site of the acetabulum, compatible with skeletal metastases (arrows). This was confirmed by needle biopsy.

was very aggressive or if clinical staging was inadequate here.

Because the reliability of clinical staging is poor for tumors in stages T2 or higher, one cannot deduce much about their overstaging with MRI compared with that with CT. Nor does the follow-up produce any increase in reliability of the clinical staging method as a reference. But in spite of this, a few statements can be made about the 24 patients with infiltrative tumors.

CT missed a stage T2 tumor or higher tumor in two patients, whereas MRI staged them correctly. The reason for this was the inability of CT to generate images in the coronal and sagittal planes or to differentiate between bladder wall hypertrophy and tumor. In four patients with tumor invasion of the prostate, the tumor could be staged as T4A by the clinical staging method. The MRI staging was correct

in all these patients. Conversely, CT gave the correct diagnosis in only one patient.

In order to obtain some insight into the staging value of MRI compared with CT in a larger group of patients, the staging results of these two techniques for all patients in this section and section 5.2 are presented in Table 23. There is a definite difference in staging by the two techniques (agreement, 50%), especially for stages (T0 and T4A) determined by MRI.

N staging

The results of lymphography combined with follow-up agree completely with those of MRI (see Table 24A and 24B). This is not surprising, as all the lymph nodes containing metastases were clearly enlarged. During CT, in two patients, blood vessels were mistaken for abnormally enlarged lymph nodes. In another patient, diseased lymph nodes could not be recognized on CT. The ability of MRI to produce images in more than one plane and to differentiate between blood vessels and lymph nodes results in a greater accuracy of MRI compared with CT. The fact that CT and MRI score equally in published reports (see also Table 7, section 1.2.5) in N staging may be because these authors primarily base their staging on transverse images. In this study, the presence of diseased lymph nodes was assessed on MRI images in three planes, the coronal plane appearing to be the most important.

M staging

When the pelvis was imaged with MRI, distant metastases were found in seven patients. In all these patients, the metastases were in the bone marrow of the lower lumbar vertebral column, in the pelvis or in the femurs. The bone marrow metastases were particularly well displayed on the STIR images and less easy to see on the T_2-weighted images (Fig. 3-8).

In accordance with the findings of other authors,[24, 49] MR would appear to be better than scintigraphy for detecting skeletal metastases: scintigraphy proved to be less sensitive than MRI in two patients. CT and conventional radiography gave an even lower score: false-negative in five and six of the seven patients, respectively.

5.3.4   Interim conclusion

The staging results of MRI and CT are diverge widely. In the 80 patients in whom both an MRI and a CT study were performed, there was only agreement in

50% of the cases. The distinction between *fibrous/ granulation/infected tissue* and *tumor* is hampered in both MRI and in CT by previous transurethral resection. However, MRI does score slightly better. As already described in Chapter 3 and section 5.2, MRI can differentiate 'late' fibrosis from tumor.

Although the value of the clinical staging method is limited as a reference for distinguishing tumors in *stages T2 and higher*, MRI appears to score better than CT. CT missed two tumors in stages T2 or higher. The determination of tumor invasion into the prostate was also a problem with CT.
MRI appeared to be equal to lymphography. However, the field of view with the sandwich coil, as used at 0.5 T, was too small for a proper determination of the N stage. CT gave a slightly worse score in the N stages than did MRI and lymphography.

Finally, MRI appears to be valuable in the recognition of bone marrow metastases.

5.4   Evaluation of MRI by using a combination of clinical staging and follow-up as a reference

In this section, the results presented are mainly those of patients with tumors staged as Ta and T1 and of patients with local fibrosis or granulation tissue resulting from transurethral resection performed much earlier (stage T0). These patients were treated with local transurethral resection, usually followed by rinsing the bladder with cytostatics or by BCG therapy. Neither CT nor lymphography were performed. As in the preceding section, the clinical staging method, backed up by follow-up was used as a reference.

Table 25   Staging results with MRI (T stages).

	clinical staging method (incl. follow-up)			
	T0	Ta-1	≥ T2	number of patients
MRI stage				
T0	**11**	2	—	
Ta-2	—	**25** (1*)	1	
≥ T3A	3	1	8*	
	——	——	——	
n	14	28	9	51

* = recurrence.

5.4.1   Patients, method and results

In 51 patients (41 men and 10 women) with UBC, an MRI study and the clinical staging method were performed.

T staging

In 19 patients, transurethral resection was performed before the MRI study and clinical staging. The interval between the earlier resection and the other two studies was at least 3 months. In these patients, there was suspicion of tumor relapse from a UBC treated much earlier with transurethral resection. In the other 32 patients, no previous transurethral resection had been performed.

The results of the MRI study are presented in Table 25. Here too, the tumors are divided into stage T0, Ta-T1, and T2 or higher, in accordance with section 5.3. The patients who suffered a relapse during the follow-up period also are indicated.

In 42 patients, by using the clinical staging method, tumors were staged as T0 (14 times) and Ta-T1 (28 times). A small superficial relapse was found only in 1 of these patients during the follow-up period.

In 3 of the 14 patients with T0 tumors, granulation and infected tissue resulting from an earlier transurethral resection was mistaken for a stage T3A tumor (once) and a stage T3B tumor (twice). In another patient with a tumor staged as Ta-T1, overstaging (stage T3B) resulted from earlier resection. Of the 28 patients with a stage Ta-T1 tumor, the tumor was not visible on MRI in one case. In another patient, the tumor had too low a signal intensity to be recognized as such on the T_2-weighted images. In 25 of the 28 patients, stage Ta-T1 tumors could be differentiated correctly.

The group of patients with tumors staged as T2 or higher was too small to allow any conclusion (9 patients).

N staging

Lymphography was not performed in any of these patients. Pathologically enlarged lymph nodes were seen on MRI in two patients, both of whom had an aggressive, infiltrative tumor.

M staging

In three patients, MRI indicated distant metastases. There was a local tumor core in all of them. The metastases were localized ventral to the urinary bladder, parailiacally, and in the penis. In the last patient, this was confirmed by biopsy.

5.4.2   Discussion

Here again, the value of the clinical staging method as reference in staging tumors in stage less than T2 (in 42 patients) is backed up by the follow-up. A small superficial relapse was found in only 1 of the 42 patients.

Differentiation between *fibrous/infected/granulation tissue (stage T0)*, resulting from an earlier transurethral resection, and tumor also posed a problem in this group of patients. In three patients, considerable overstaging occurred. However, in this group, the other MRI results were not unfavourable: staging was correct in 11 of the 14 patients.

Staging results with MRI in the patients with a *stage Ta-T1* tumor were good: the diagnosis was correct in 25 of the 28 patients. Only two tumors smaller than 5 mm were missed. Considering the small number of patients with tumors in stage T2 or higher and the lack of dependability of the reference for this stage, no reliable statement can be made about the value of MRI for these stages.

N staging

Lymphography was not performed in this group.

M staging

MRI revealed distant metastases in three patients.

5.4.3   Interim conclusion

This group supplements the previous one (sections 5.2 and 5.3). It mainly deals with patients without residual tumors and patients with stage Ta-T1 tumors. One thing was very noticeable: MRI staged tumors well in patients with tumors in stages Ta-T1. Also, the distinction between fibrous/infected/granulation tissue (stage T0), resulting from an earlier resection, and tumor was reasonable. Overstaging did, however, occur in three patients. MRI also was useful in tracing local distant metastases.

VI

DISCUSSION, CONCLUSIONS
AND FUTURE PROSPECTS

6.1 Discussion and conclusions

On the basis of the results presented in Chapters 2-5, we will try to answer the questions posed in section 1.4:

1. *Which is the best MR technique for imaging the urinary bladder?*

For the best imaging of the urinary bladder, images must be made in three different planes. Preferably, these are the coronal, sagittal, and transverse planes. It is best to use a T_1-weighted sequence.
A T_2-weighted sequence is necessary for determining the depth of invasion of the tumour into the bladder wall and for differentiating between late fibrosis, hematoma, and tumor.

At both 0.5 T and at 1.5 T, the best T_1-weighted sequence is SE/750/30/2. The best T_2-weighted sequence at 0.5 T is SE/2100/30,150/2 and at 1.5 T is SE/2100/30,100/2. These results concur with those of other authors (see Table 9).

The use of the STIR sequence (IR/2000/225/ $\leq$ 60/2) for imaging UBC has not yet been described. An advantage of this sequence is that the fat signal can be suppressed and that T_1 and T_2 effects supplement each other. The result is a very high signal intensity for infected and tumors, meaning they are easily differentiated from other tissues. This is particularly important for showing bone marrow metastases.

Use of a double surface coil at a field strength of 0.5 T results in considerable improvement in image quality and hence an increase in staging accuracy. An optimal double surface coil for 1.5 T is not readily available; however, the results with a less than optimal version are encouraging.
Staging of invasive tumors at a field strength of 1.5 T *without* a surface coil is equivalent to that at 0.5 T *with* a surface coil. The larger field of view of the images made at 1.5 T without surface coil allows better recognition of metastases. As the value of MRI mainly resides in the staging of invasive UBC s (see question 4), preference is given to a field strength of 1.5 T.

2. *How does MRI display the normal anatomy of the urinary bladder?*

Thanks to excellent tissue contrast, images in several planes and the lack of interfering respiratory artifacts, the relationship between the urinary bladder and surrounding organs can be well displayed. Because of their low signal intensity, blood vessels can be differentiated from other structures without use of contrast agents.

MR images of patients without pelvic abnormalities and of anatomical material suggest MR imaging depicts the anatomic substrate accurately.

3. *How does MRI display tumors of the urinary bladder?*

The morphology of UBC can be recognized on T_1-weighted images, as it can on CT scans. In general, on T_2-weighted images, the tumor has a higher signal intensity than does normal bladder wall or fibrosis. The differentiation between tumor and normal bladder wall or fibrosis can be hampered by motion artifacts or by an abnormally high signal intensity of the bladder wall. The latter mainly occurs after a transurethral resection, after radiotherapy or because of cystitis.

Lymph node metastases are recognized by their abnormal size and not because of an abnormal signal intensity. This has been found by other authors also.[57] Bone marrow metastases can be seen as an area of signal intensity resembling that of a primary tumor of the urinary bladder. The signal intensity is low on T_1-weighted images, high on T_2-weighted images and very high on STIR sequences.

4. *What is the value of MRI with respect to the UBC?*

When evaluating an investigative technique, three concepts must be distinguished:

1. *eficiency*: this indicates the value of the investigative technique for establishing the diagnosis. It can be the value of the technique for detecting a certain abnormality (*detection value*) or the value is the value of the investigative technique in determining the extent of the abnormality (*staging value*).

2. *efficacy*: this indicates the usefulness of the investigative technique for a specific purpose (e.g., treatment).

3. *effectiveness*: this indicates the effectiveness of the combination of the investigative technique and therapy.

In evaluating the use of MRI in UBC, efficiency was analysed first. The *staging value* is particularly important here, because the high costs associated with MRI make it unsuitable for use in detecting UBC.

When the staging value of MRI is assessed, one also must consider its usefulness from a therapeutic point of view. It is important to establish whether MRI can supplement existing staging procedures and which of these can be omitted by use of MRI. Determining the effectiveness (technology assessment) is beyond the scope of this book. Not only the diagnostic investigative technique must be assessed, but also the value of a certain form of treatment. Reliable information on this issue can be obtained only after a very long follow-up period and epidemiologic study. The follow-up period for the patients described in the this study is far too short and the numbers too small to allow conclusions to be drawn. Furthermore, the results of the MRI examinations were not integrated into the therapeutic policy.

MRI versus the clinical staging method

Compared with the clinical staging method, the accuracy of MRI in staging tumors as T3A or more is significantly higher (p $<$ .01, McNemar test). On the other hand, however, it is the clinical staging method that can distinguish between stages Ta-T1 and T2, not MRI.

The clinical staging method also is more reliable in determining the presence or absence of a tumor after a transurethral resection. This differentiation is problematic with MRI: in 12 (15%) of the 78 patients the tumor was overstaged. In 4 patients, granulation and infected tissues ware mistakenly interpreted as a deeply infiltrated tumor.

MRI is very capable of determining the N and M stages, something that is difficult to achieve with the clinical staging method. The staging results for the N stages obtained with MRI are certainly no worse, and may well be better than, those with lymphography. Compared with results reported elsewhere (Table 6),

lymphography scores slightly lower in the present study. The MRI staging results agree with those of other authors (see Table 7). None of these authors, however, compare the results of MRI with those of lymphography.

The results in a few patients appear to indicate that MRI has certain advantages over scintigraphy and conventional radiographic studies in establishing the presence of bone marrow metastases. This book may act as a stimulus for further research in this direction. The present study does not support the opinion of other researchers that MRI has low specificity for bone marrow metastases (H.Hricak, personal communication 1988).

MRI versus CT

MRI is more accurate than CT in determining T stages. The degree of overstaging and understaging with CT is definitely larger than with MRI. This is also found by other authors (see Table 7). The only area in which no significant difference is seen between these techniques is the distinction between stages T3A and T3B.

In accord with the experience of other investigators (Table 7), T staging in patients who had undergone transurethral resection was mediocre with both MRI and CT. MRI overstaged tumors in 12 (15%) of the 78 patients. With CT, tumors were overstaged in 14 (25%) of the 56 patients. Both techniques produced considerable overstaging in 4 patients: infected and granulation tissues were mistaken for an invasive tumor. The reason for this high percentage of overstaging is the inability of either technique to distinguish infected tissue from tumor tissue. The difference between MRI and CT lies in MRI's ability to differentiate between fibrosis and tumor.

The staging of the N stages is better with MRI, although published reports (see Table 7, section 1.2.5) indicate that CT and MRI score equally; this could be because these authors mainly base their tumor staging on transverse images. In this study, the presence of diseased lymph nodes is assessed on MR images made in three planes, the coronal plane proving to be the most important.

Although only a small number of patients had distant metastases in the pelvic region, MRI also ap-

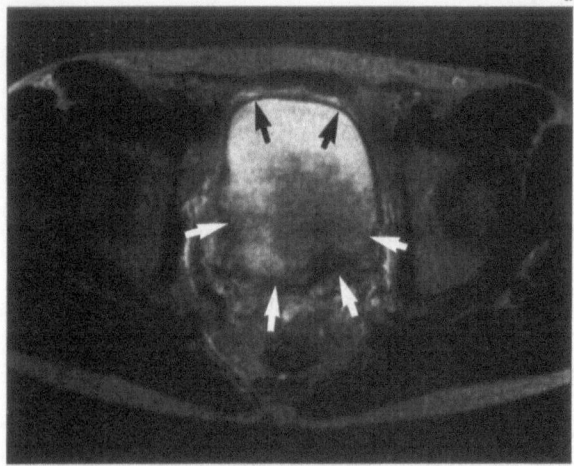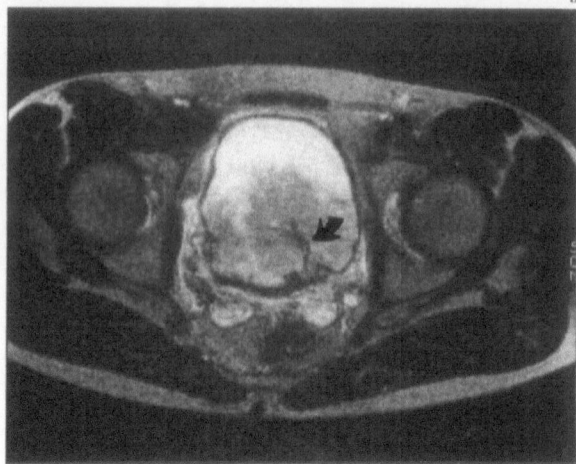

Fig. 6-1. (a) The MR image made before chemotherapy reveals an interruption (white arrows) of the normal urinary bladder wall (black arrows) (at least stage T3A). **(b)** MR image made after chemotherapy shows a normal low-signal bladder wall, compatible with a decrease in tumor infiltration (stage Ta-T2). This was confirmed on histologic examination the resected specimen (stage T1). The vascular peduncle in the tumor (curved arrow) can be seen on **(b)**.

pears to have certain advantages compared with CT for determining the M stage. MRI was better for recognizing peritonitis carcinomatosa, local metastases, and bone marrow metastases. To date, no reports have been published concerning the MRI visualization of such metastasis at a distance from the UBC.

5. *Can MRI replace other, existing staging techniques?*

When answering this question, one should consider not only the efficiency, but also the efficacy of MRI. A key question is of what benefit is the improved staging obtained with MRI to the therapy to be initiated? The answer to this question depends on the local therapeutic policy (see section 1.2.1). Before one can delineate this policy, one must

a. determine the histopathologic staging,
b. differentiate between stages Ta-T1 and T2. Cystectomy is not performed, nor is radiotherapy used in patients with a stage Ta-T1 tumor. Conversely, in patients in whom the tumor infiltrates the muscle wall (stage T2), such forms of therapy are used.
c. determine the depth of growth if the tumor does penetrate the perivesical fat. If invasion is limited, curative cystectomy or radiotherapy is performed. If there is deep invasion into the fat, the only choice is palliative therapy.
d. differentiate between stages T3B and T4A/T4B. If there is invasion of nearby organs (stage T4A)

or of the pelvic cavity or abdominal wall (stage T4B), palliative therapy must suffice. In cases where there is growth into the uterus, vagina, or prostate (stage T4A), an attempt is made to achieve a cure by means of radical resection.
e. find out whether metastases are present. If this is the case, curative therapy is not even considered. An attempt is made to achieve palliation by means of chemotherapy.
f. finally, monitor the effects of chemotherapeutics.[200, 209, 211, 224, 233] It is important to be able to quantify accurately any tumor regression that might occur. It is especially important to establish whether a tumor of a stage that would be treated palliatively decreases to a stage that can be cured (Fig. 6-1).

Histopathologic staging is part of the clinical staging method. Histologic information cannot be obtained with CT or MRI.
The clinical staging method is clearly more reliable in differentiating between infected/granulation tissue, resulting from earlier transurethral resection, and tumor. Overstaging occurs with both MRI and CT, in 15% and 25% of patients, respectively. Even considerable overstaging -infected and granulation tissue being mistaken for a deeply infiltrated tumor- is found in 5% with MRI and 7% with CT. The clinical staging method is the most reliable for differentiating between tumors staged as Ta-T1 and T2.
MRI is the best technique for determining the degree of tumor growth into the muscle layer (differentia-

tion between stages T2 and T3A). If MRI is used, very deep transurethral resection is no longer required for this differentiation. Furthermore, MRI is the most reliable technique for determining tumor penetration into the perivesical fat and for the staging of tumors as T3B, T4A, and T4B.

The determination of lymph node metastases is certainly no worse with MRI than with CT or lymphography. The results of staging with MRI are possibly even somewhat better. As this MRI study only portrayed nodes in the lower abdomen, no statement can be made about lymph nodes in the upper abdomen. However, in all patients in this study, lymph node metastasis was first noticed in the pelvis. MRI missed only micrometastases in nonenlarged lymph nodes; other techniques also failed to detect these. Lymphography appears to be indicated only if MRI produces a dubious result regarding lymph node metastasis.

Finally, MRI would seem to be the best imaging technique for detecting distant metastases in the pelvis.

Recommendations:

If the MRI facilities are limited, it is not recommended that all patients with UBC undergo MRI. Only those patients in whom the clinical staging method shows at least minimal tumor invasion of the muscle layer (stage T2 or higher) should be considered for MRI. One must simply accept serious overstaging, which only occurs in 5% of the patients. In any case, this percentage lower than that obtained with CT (7% of patients). The strategy recommended for examining patients with a UBC is therefore:

a. *first*, use the *clinical staging method*. If there is any invasion of the muscle layer (stage T2 or higher),
b. an *MRI examination should be performed*;
c. *CT can be omitted*;
d. MRI need be followed by *lymphography* only in *dubious* cases of lymph node metastasis.

6.2 Future prospects

As we did not have our own MRI equipment, we could not make optimal use of MR contrast agents or of the newest MRI techniques. A few points that seem to be highly promising in the future of MRI of the UBC are briefly expounded on in the following sections.

6.2.1 Surface coils

New double surface coils, better than the one used in the present study, have been developed for magnetic fields of 1.5 T. They allow one to vary the size of the field to be displayed. These coils result in a better quality of image than possible with the surface coil used here, and hence are bound to improve the staging results of UBC. Intrarectal surface coils also have been described.

6.2.2 Contrast agents

Shortly after the development of MRI, the superfluity of contrast media was named as one of the advantages of this technique. It would always be possible to choose pulse sequences that could differentiate the various tissues.

Now it seems that, although many pulse sequences are used, MRI has a high sensitivity for showing various diseases, but its specificity is disappointing. The future development of tissue-, organ-, and tumor-specific MR contrast agents will surely be an improvement.[154,185] Another potential use for such substances could be the measurement of organ perfusion at the capillary level.[47]
A thorough description of the action of these MR contrast agents is beyond the scope of this book. The reader is, therefore, referred to the literature.[16, 29, 33, 46, 47, 53, 71, 136, 154, 185, 194-196, 230]

Two groups of contrast media that could be of interest in staging UBC are
a. those that can be administered *orally* and
b. those that can be administered *intravenously*.

Tumour tissue cannot be differentiated from the intestine on the basis of signal intensity on MRI images. The use of *orally* administered contrast media, which alter the signal intensity of the intestine, will enable better distinction of tumor tissue. This is particularly important when determining tumor growth into the intestine itself (stage T4A), when dilineating abnormally enlarged lymph nodes and when determining lymphangitis carcinomatosa. Oral contrast media are currently being used only experimentally.

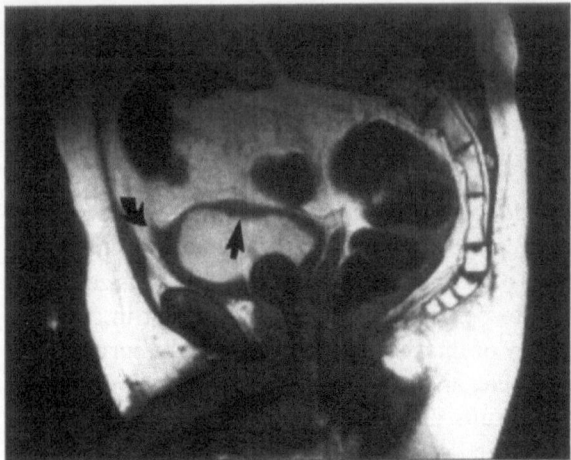

Fig. 6-2. Sagittal MR image (SE/750/30/2) after intravenous injection of 4 ml Gd-DTPA. Because of the fine staining of the urinary bladder lumen, the wall can be assessed very accurately: thick bladder floor and thickening at the bladder roof (arrow). The median umbilical ligament can be seen ventrally (curved arrow). The lumen of the bladder catheter also is stained.

Gd-DTPA is the main constituent of *intravenous* MR contrast media (Magnevist, Schering). This substance has a very strong T_1-reducing effect and, therefore, results in a very high signal on T_1-weighted images. The Gd-DTPA is excreted via the kidneys and, even at a low dosage (2 ml intravenous), produces a very high signal in the urine on T_1-weighted images. As in the administration of contrast agents in CT,[4, 90, 91, 102, 161, 167, 197, 234] this can result in better recognition and staging of small UBCs (Figs. 6-2 and 6-3). From images of the kidneys, one also can draw conclusions about kidney function and urine flow via the ureters.

It is still not clear whether UBC has a different stain than the bladder wall itself. If the tumor had a higher signal intensity, this would increase discrimination between it and the bladder wall. Further research into these contrast agents is needed.

6.2.3   Fast sequences

By reducing the initial 90 rotation of the magnetization axis of the protons (see Chapter 2), it is possible to reduce TR and TE and thus to shorten considerably the imaging time. In this way, with a 128 x 128 matrix, one image can be generated in 3 sec. Various names are applied to these fast imaging techniques: FFE, FLASH, FISP, or GRASS (see also section 3.2.2).[77, 78, 158, 170] With these sequences, it is possible to generate an image that resembles a T_2-weighted image, (T_2*-weighted image) within a very short time.

Varying the angle of rotation (flip-angle) produces a great change in image contrast. At a small flip-angle (15), a T_2* weighted image emerges (Fig. 6-4). At a flip-angle of 60°-90°, the image is T_1 weighted (Fig. 6-5). On the other hand, changes in TR and TE do not have much effect on the image contrast.

Three-dimensional (3-D) images also can be prepared with this sequence.[127, 193] The advantage of this 3-D technique is that one can obtain images in any plane within a period of 5-10 min. Disadvantages of the fast sequences are

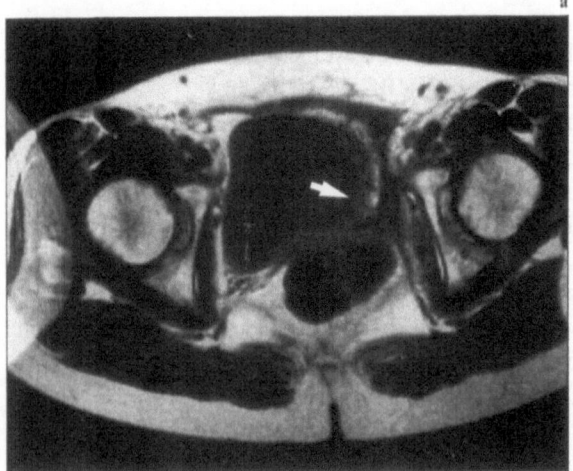
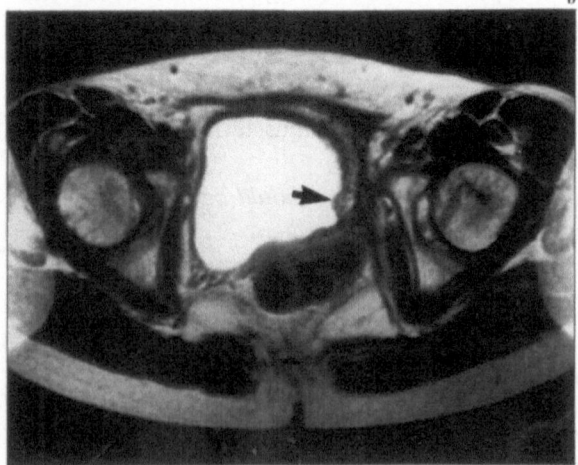

Fig. 6-3. (a) The transverse MR image (1.5 T; SE/800/30/2) reveals local thickening of the bladder wall on the left side (arrow). **(b)** This can, however, be assessed much better after intravenous injection of 2 ml Gd-DTPA (same acquisition parameters).

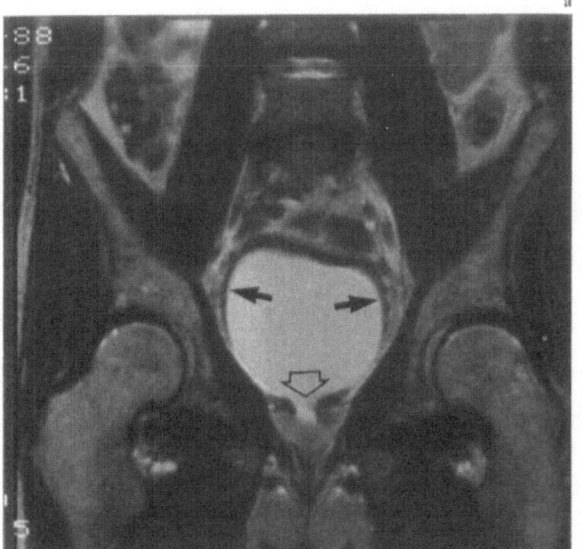
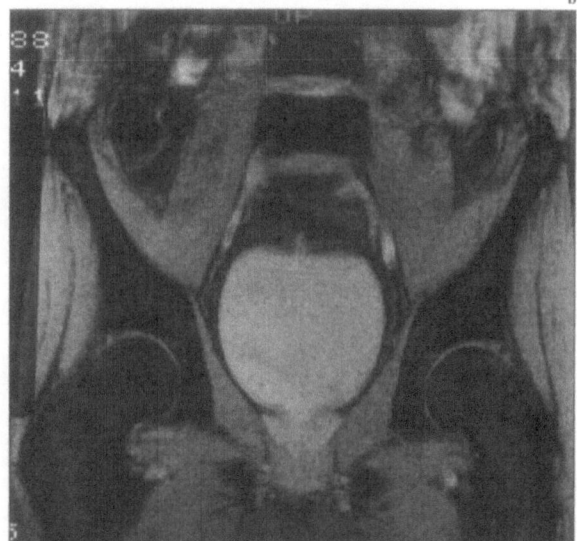

Fig. 6-4. Coronal MR images: **(a)** T2-weighted image (1.5 T; SE/2000/90/2) and **(b)** T2*weighted image (1.5 T; FISP/150/15/2, α = 15) (see also Fig. 4-1).

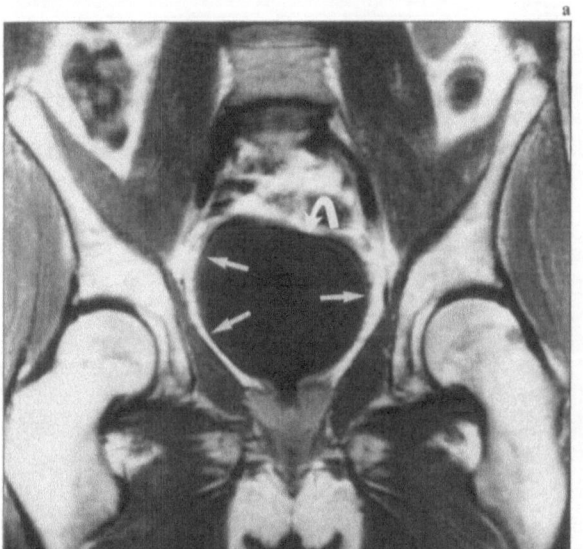
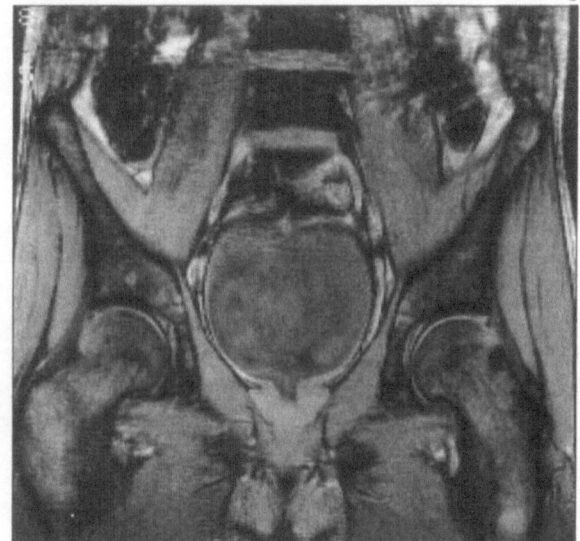

Fig. 6-5. Coronal MR images: **(a)** T1-weighted image (1.5 T;SE/1000/15/2) and **(b)** FISP/150/12/2, α = 70 (see also Fig. 4-1).

a. The high sensitivity to movement. When generating images of the urinary bladder, the effects of bladder movement and of intestinal peristalsis in particular are intensified.

b. The T_2 contrast is not as good as that on a T_2-weighted SE image. Accordingly, one refers to a T_2*weighted sequence.

c. These sequences are extremely flow sensitive, resulting in enhancement of flow artifacts. On these sequences, flow of urine into the bladder also can produce artifacts.

To date, there are no published descriptions of the use of fast sequences for UBC imaging. Our first personal experience (four patients) varied: in two patients, interfering artifacts occurred because of bladder movements, inflow of urine, and intestinal peristalsis. In the two other patients, however, the imaging quality was excellent. The image quality of the fast T_2*weighted FLASH sequence in these patients was just as good as that of a T_2-weighted SE sequence (Fig. 6-4). The FLASH sequence was made in 5 min, the SE sequence in 17 min. All in all, the first results with these fast sequences seem very promising.

VII

SUMMARY

Since the introduction of magnetic resonance imaging (MRI) in the early 1980s, interest has grown in its use to stage tumors of the urinary bladder and the lower pelvic cavity.

As MRI is based on completely different physical principles than are other imaging methods, a better and alternativ differentiation between tumor and adjacent tissue can be expected. Assessment of this differentiation and determination of the value of MRI in staging carcinoma of the urinary bladder is the aim of this study.

In chapter 1, a general introduction to MRI is given. The reported efficacies of clinical staging, ultrasonography, lymphography, CT, and MRI are presented. MRI proves to be a valuable addition to the clinical staging method, but literature covering this particular field is scarce.

Chapter 2 deals with general principles of MR imaging only asextensively as is necessary to understand the following chapters.
Concepts such as T_1, and T_2 relaxation times, proton density, TR, TE and TI are discussed. Mutual relationships between these concepts and their effects on the eventual imaging are discussed in greater detail. Particular attention is paid to the most frequently used techniques, such as spin echo- and inversion recovery sequences. Generation of image contrast and artifacts, either when using astrong (1.5 T) or a weaker (0.5 T) magnetic field, are dealt with. Advantages and disadvantages of MRI are presented: MRI is a noninvasive technique that makes imaging of the human body possiblein any plane, with differentiation between various kinds of tissue. No efforts is required of the patients, and side effects are (as yet) unknown. MRI, however, is a time-consuming and expensive imaging technique. Because of the magnetic forces involved, patients with pacemakers, ferromagnetic clips (especially cerebral) and certaintypes of heart-valve prostheses are should not undergo MRI examination.

Based on published data, **in chapter 3**, the choice of the best pulse sequences is presented. For imaging carcinoma of the urinary bladder, a T_1-weighted SE sequence is best for delineating tumor from (perivesical) fat, whereas a T_2-weighted SE sequence is best for differentiating between tumor, its extent into the bladder wall, and secondary fibrosis.
Pulse sequence optimization in this study was determined by using contrast matrices and illustrated by synthetic imaging. Compared with other reports, the results of pulse sequence optimization conform well, but in this study, a short-TI inversion recovery pulse sequence was found to be very useful in detecting metastases in lymph nodes and bone marrow.
Use of a double surface coil is combination with a fieldstrength of 0.5 T resulted in significantly improved image quality. A prototype surface coil for 1.5-T field strength did not improve the image quality. Research for a better surfacecoil is underway.
The better image quality of 0.5-T field strength in combination with a double surface coil, compared withthat of 1.5 T without a surface coil, resulted in more accurate staging of superficial tumors. The staging results for deeper infiltrating tumors, however, are equal. Owing to the larger field of view with 1.5 T, more bone marrow and lymph node metastases could be detected.

Chapter 4 presents an atlas of comparative anatomy. MR images of normal volunteers are compared with MR images of an autopsy specimen and the corresponding cryosections of that specimen. Also a comparison of images of bladder tumors in vivo and after resection in vitro is presented, together with their corresponding resected specimens.

In chapter 5 the results of the various staging methods in 134 patients with carcinoma of the bladder are presented. The material is divided into three groups.
In the first group of 40 patients, the results of cystectomy are compared with results of the clinical staging method, CT, lymphography, and MRI.
In the second group of 43 patients, the clinical staging method is compared with CT, lymphography, and MRI.
The last group (51 patients) deals with comparison of the clinical staging method with MRI. In the last two groups the results of follow-up, lasting from 6 months up to 3 years, are incorporated.

MRI proves to be significantly more accurate than CT for T staging except for the T3A and T3B stages, for which both methods have the same score. As the number of patients with lymph node metastases in this study is low, a comparison of MR staging with the other staging systems is limited. MR seems to have advantages over CT scanning and lymphography in this respect. MRI also seems to have advantages for diagnosing peritonitis carcinomatosa and bone marrow metastases. Differentiation between fibrosis as a result of earlier transurethral resection and carcinoma is clearer with MRI than with CT. The clinical staging method is less accurate in differentiating between the various stages of deeper infiltrating tumors (higher than stage T2) than MRI, but more accurate in more superficial tumors (stages Ta-T1 and T2). The conclusion is that MRI and clinical staging supplement each other.

In the last chapter, **chapter 6**, the aim and the scope of the study is summarized and recommendations are made. From this study, it can be concluded that:

1. the staging of patients with carcinoma of the urinary bladder has to start with the *clinical staging method*,
2. should be followed by *MRI*, especially in *muscular wall or deeper infiltration*,
3. *CT* in staging bladder tumors *is superfluous*, and finally
4. *lymphography* is only indicated if there is any *doubt* about lymph node metastases.

REFERENCES

1. **Abu-Yousef MM,** Narayana AS, Franken EA, Brown RC. Urinary bladder tumors studied by cystosonography. Radiology 1984; 153:223-226.

2. **Adair RE,** Berglund LG. On the thermoregulatory consequences of NMR imaging. Magn Res Imag 1986; 4:321-325.

3. **Adams DF.** Biological effect and potential hazards of nuclear magnetic resonance imaging. Cardiovasc Intervent Radiol 1986; 8:260-263.

4. **Ahlberg NE,** Calissendorff B, Wijkström H. Computed tomography in staging of bladder carcinoma. Acta Radiol Diagn 1982; 23:47-53.

5. **Alzin HH,** Brädel HU, Schwaiger R, Kopper B. Vergleich zwischen Computertomogramm und endovesikaler Sonographie bei der Diagnostik und Klassifikation grosserer Blasentumoren. Verh dt Ges Urol 1983; 35:231-233.

6. **Amendola MA,** Glaser GM, Grossman HB, et al. Staging of bladder carcinoma: MRI-CT-surgical correlation. AJR 1986; 146:1179-1183.

7. **Arsonval MA.** Dispositifs pour la mesure des courants alternatifs a toutes frequences. Cr Soc Biol 1986; 3:451-454.

8. **Bakker CJG.** Some exercises in quantitative NMR imaging. Proefschrift 1985 Utrecht, Drukkerij Elinkwijk BV.

9. **Bangert V,** Mansfield P. Whole-body tomographic imaging by NMR. Br J Radiol 1981; 54:152-154.

10. **Barentsz JO,** Lemmens JAM, Boskamp EB et al. Improved MR imaging of the bladder by using a new surface coil. Fortschr Röntgenstr 1986; 145:351-353.

11. **Barentsz JO,** Lemmens JAM, Ruijs SHJ et al. Carcinoma of the urinary bladder: MR imaging using a double surface coil. AJR 1988; 151:107-112.

12. **Barentsz JO,** Ruijs JHJ, Heystraten FMJ, Buskens F. Magnetic resonance of the dissected thoracic aorta. Br J Radiol 1987; 60:499-502.

13. **Barentsz JO,** Ruijs JHJ, Karthaus HFM et al. Mogelijkheden van kernspinresonantie-tomografie bij maligne tumoren van de urineblaas. Ned Tijdschr voor Geneesk 1987; 131:2190-2194.

14. **Bartels KD,** Dettmar H, Göckel B. Die Bedeutung der Computertomographie bei der Stadieneinteilung der Harnblasentumoren. Urologe 1983; 22:342-346.

15. **Bassett CAL,** Pilla AA, Pawluk RJ. A non-operative salvage of surgical resistant pseudarthroses and non-unions by pulsating electromagnetic fields. Clin Orthop 1977; 124:128-131.

16. **Bell R.** An overview for contrast agents for magnetic resonance imaging. Book of abstracts 6th SMRM 1987:110-112.

17. **Bellon EM,** Haacke EM, Coleman PE et al. MR artifacts: a review. AJR 1986; 147:1271-1281.

18. **Bergman SM,** Lippert M, Javadpour N. The value of whole lung tomography in the early detection of metastatic disease in patients with renal cell carcinoma and testicular tumors. J. Urol 1980; 124:860-862.

19. **Bernardino ME,** Thomas JL, Barnes PA, Lewis E. Diagnostic approaches to liver and spleen metastases. Rad Clin N Am 1982; 20:469-472.

20. **Beyer HK,** Funke PJ, Brackins-Romero J, Ühlenbrock D. Wertigkeit der Kernspintomographie bei der Diagnostik und Stadienbestimmung von Harnblasenneoplasmen. Digit Bilddiagnost 1985; 5:167-172.

21. **Bezzi M,** Kressel HY, Allen KS, et al. Prostatic carcinoma: staging with MR imaging at 1.5 T. Radiology 1988; 169:339-346.

22. **Bloch F,** Hansen WW, Packard M. Nuclear induction. Phys Rev 1946; 69:127-129.

23. **Bloch F.** Nuclear induction. Phys Rev 1946; 70:460-474.

24. **Bloem JL.** Radiological staging of primary malignant musculoskeletal tumors. A correlative study of CT, MRI, 99mTC scintigraphy and angiography. Proefschrift 1988 Den Haag.

25. **Bondestam S,** Laehde S, Annala RA, et al. Scintigraphy and sonography in the investigation of liver metastases. Diagnostic Imaging 1980; 49: 339-343.

26. **Boskamp EB.** Improved surface coil imaging in MR: decoupling of the excitation and receiver coils. Radiology 1985; 157:449-452.

27. **Bottomley PA.** In vivo tumor discrimination in a rat by proton nuclear magnetic resonance. Cancer Research 1979; 39:468-470.

28. **Bottomley PA,** Foster TH, Argersinger RE, Pfeifer LM. A review of normal tissue hydrogen NMR relaxation times and relaxation mechanisms from 1-100 MHz: dependence on tissue type, NMR frequency, temperature, species, excision and age. Med Phys 1984; 11:425-448.

29. **Bousquet JC,** Saini S, Stark DD et al. Gd-DTPA: Characterization of a new paramagnetic complex. Radiology 1988; 166:693-698.

30. **Bradley WG.** Flow phenomena. In: Stark DD, Bradley WG eds. Magnetic resonance imaging 1988; 108-137. St Louis, Mosby.

31. **Bradley WG.** Flow phenomena. In: Syllabus: a categorical course in diagnostic radiology. MR imaging. Stark DD, Bradley WG, eds. 74th RSNA meeting 1988:27-37.

32. **Braeckman J,** Denis L. The practice and pittfalls of ultrasonography in the lower urinary tract. Eur Urol 1983; 9:193-201.

33. **Brash RC en Bennet HF.** Considerations in the choice of contrast media for MR Imaging. Radiology 1988; 166:897-899.

34. **Bryan BJ,** Butler HE, LiPuma JP, et al. NMR scanning of the pelvis: initial experience with a 0.3 T system. AJR 1983; 141:1111-1118.

35. **Bryan PJ,** Butler HE, LiPuma JP et al. CT and MR imaging in staging bladder neoplasms. J Comp Ass Tom 1987; 11:96-101.

36. **Bryan PJ,** Dinn WM, Grossman ZD, et al. Correlation of computed tomography, gray scale ultrasonography and radionuclide imaging of the liver in detection space-occupying processes. Radiology 1979; 130:201-205.

37. **Buchli R,** Bösiger P, Meier D. Heating effects of metallic implants by MRI examinations. Magn Res in Med 1988; 7:255-261.

38. **Budinger TF.** Thresholds for physiological effects due to RF and magnetic fields used in NMR Imaging. IEEE Trans Nucl Sci NS 1979; 26:2821-2825.

39. **Budinger TF.** Saftey of NMR in vivo imaging and spectroscopy. In: Medical magnetic resonance imaging and spectroscopy. Budinger TF, Marguilis AR (eds). Soc of magn res in Med Berkeley, CA 1986:215-233.

40. **Budinger TF,** Cullander C. Health effecs of in vivo magnetic resonance. In: Clinical magnetic resonance imaging. Marguilis AR, Higgins CB, Kaufman L, Crooks LE (eds), Radiol. Res. & Educ. Found. 1983, S.Francisco.

41. **Bureau of radiological health:** guide-lines for evaluating electromagnetic exposure risk for trials and clinical NMR systems, Washington DC: Dept of Health and Human Services, US Public Health Service, Food and Drug Administration, 1982.

42. **Butler H,** Bryan PJ, LiPuma PJ et al. Magnetic resonance imaging of the abnormal female pelvis. AJR 1984; 143:1259-1266.

43. **Buy JN**, Moss AA, Guinet C et al. MR staging of bladder carcinoma: correlation with pathologic findings. Radiology 1988; 169:695-700.

44. **Bydder GM**, Steiner RE, Blumgart LH et al. MR imaging of the liver using short TI inversion recovery sequences. J Comp Ass Tom 1985; 9:1084-1089.

45. **Bydder GM**, Young IR. MR imaging: clinical use of the inversion recovery sequence. J Comp Ass Tom 1985; 9:659-675.

46. **Carr DH**, Brown J, Bydder GM et al. Intravenous chelated gadolinium as a contrast agent in NMR imaging in cerebral tumors. Lancet 1984; 1:484-486.

47. **Carr DH**. The use of proton relaxation enhancers in magnetic resonance imaging. Magn Res Imag 1985; 3:17-25.

48. **Chang YCF**, Hricak H, Thurnher S, Lacey CG. Vagina: evaluation with MR imaging. Part II. Neoplasms. Radiology 1988; 169:175-179.

49. **Daffner RH**, Lupetin AR, Dash et al. MRI in the detection of malignant infiltration of bòne marrow. AJR 1986;146:353-361.

50. **Damadian R.** Tumor detection by nuclear magnetic resonance. Science 1971; 171:1151-1153.

51. **Davey P**, Merrick MV, Duncan W, Redpath AT. Bladder cancer: the value of routine bone scintigraphy. Clin Radiology 1985; 36:77-79.

52. **Davis PL**, Crooks L, Arakawa M et al. Potential hazards in NMR imaging: heating effects of changing magnetic fields and RF fields on small metallic implants. AJR 1981; 137:857-861.

53. **Davis PL**, Parker DL, Nelson JA et al. Interaction of paramagnetic contrast agents and the spin echo pulse sequence. Invest Radiol 1988; 23:381-388.

54. **Degani H**, Horowitz A, Itzchak Y. Phosphorus-31 magnetic resonance studies of human breast tumors. RSNA '85 'Work in Progress' 1985.

55. **Demas BE**, Hricak H, Gore J. Uterine MR imaging effects of hormonal stimulation. Radiology 1986; 159:123-126.

56. **Denkhaus H**, Crone-Muenzebrock W, Huland H. Noninvasive ultrasound in detecting and staging bladder carcinoma. Urol Radiol 1985; 7:121-131.

57. **Dooms GC**, Hricak H, Crooks LE, Higgins CB. Magnetic resonance imaging of lymph nodes: comparison with CT. Radiology 1984; 153:719-728.

58. **Dooms GC**, Hricak H, Tscholakoff D. Adnexal structures: MR imaging. Radiology 1986; 158:639-644.

59. **Dunnick NR**, Javadpour N. Value of CT and lymphography: distinguishing retroperitoneal metastases from non-seminomatous testicular tumors. AJR 1981; 137:207-211.

60. **Dunnill MS**, Anderson JA, Whitehead R. Quantitative histological studies on age changes in bone. J Pathol Bacteriol 1967; 94:,275-291.

61. **Dwyer AJ**, Frank JA, Sank VJ et al. Short-TI-Inversion-Recovery pulse sequence: analysis and initial experience in cancer imaging. Radiology 1988; 168:827-836.

62. **Ebner F**, Kressel HY, Mintz MC et al. Tumor recurrence versus fibrosis in the female pelvis: differentiation with MR imaging at 1.5 T. Radiology 1988; 166:333-340.

63. **Edelman RR**, McFarland E, Stark DD. Surface coil MR imaging of the abdominal viscera. Part I. Theory, technique and initial results. Radiology 1985; 157:425-430.

64. **Edelstein WA**, Bottomley PA, Hart HR, Smith LS. Signal, noise and contrast in nuclear magnetic resonance (NMR) imaging. J Comp Ass Tom 1983; 7:391-401.

65. **Edelstein WA**, Hutchison JMS, Smith FW, et al. Human whole-body NMR tomographic imaging: normal sections. Br J Radiol 1981; 54:149-151.

66. **Ehman RL.** MR imaging with surface coils. Radiology 1985; 157:549-550.

67. **Engelmann U**, Schild H, Klose K, et al. Die Treffsicherheit der Computertomographie beim Harnblasenkarzinom. Urologe 1984; 23:161-166.

68. **Essed E**, Boon ME, Donker PJ. Blaaskanker: stagering en behandeling. Ned Tijdschr voor Geneesk 1980; 124:786-792.

69. **Farrar TC**, Becker ED. Pulse and fourier transform NMR. 1971 New York, Academic Press.

70. **Feinberg DA**, Mills CM, Posin JP, et al. Multiple spin echo magnetic resonance imaging. Radiology 1985; 155:437-442.

71. **Felix R**, Semmler W, Schörner W en Laniado M. Contrast media for magnetic resonance tomography. Fortschr Röntgenstr 1985; 142:641-646.

72. **Feuerbach S**, Rupp N, Rossmann W et al. Lymphknotenmetastasen - Diagnose durch Lymphographie und CT. Forschr Röntgenstr 1979; 130:323-328.

73. **Finn EJ**, Di Chiro G, Brooks RA, et al. Ferromagnetic materials in patients: detection before MR imaging. Radiology 1985; 156:139-141.

74. **Fisher MR**, Barker B, Amparo EG. MR imaging using specialised coils. Radiology 1985; 157:443-447.

75. **Fisher MR**, Hricak H, Crooks LE. Urinary bladder MR imaging. Part I. Normal and benign conditions. Radiology 1985; 157:467-470.

76. **Fisher MR**, Hricak H, Tanagho EA. Urinary bladder MR imaging. Part II. Neoplasm. Radiology 1985; 157:471-477.

77. **Frahm J**, Haase A, Matthaei D. Rapid MR imaging using the FLASH technique. J Com Ass Tomogr 1986; 10:363-368.

78. **Frahm, J**, Haasse A, Matthaei D. Rapid NMR imaging of dynamic processes using the FLASH technique. Magn Reson Med 1986; 3:321-327.

79. **Fritzsche PJ.** Male pelvis. In: Syllabus: a categorical course in diagnostic radiology. MR imaging. Stark DD, Bradley WG, eds. 74th RSNA meeting 1988:149-154.

80. **Frödin L**, Hemmingson A, Johansson A, Wicklund H. Computed tomography in staging of bladder carcinoma. Acta Radiol Diagn 1980; 21:763-767.

81. **Fullerton GD**, Cameron IL, Ord VA. Frequency dependence of magnetic resonance spin-lattice relaxation of protons in biological materials. Radiology 1984; 151:135-138.

82. **Gaffey CT**, Tenforde TS. Bioelectric properties of frog sciatic nerves during exposure to static magnetic fields. Radiat Environ Biophys 1983; 22:61-65.

83. **Geacintov NE**, Nostrand F van, Becker JF et al. Magnetic field induced orientation of photosynthetic systems. Biochem Biophys Acta 1972; 262:65-69.

84. **Gelfand DW**, Ott DJ. Methodologic considerations in comparing imaging methods. AJR 1985; 144:1117-1121.

85. **Greiner KG**, Jacob F, Klose KC, Schwartz R. Sicherung der T-Klassifikation von Harnblasentumoren durch transkutane Sonographie, intravesikale Sonographie und Computertomographie. Fortschr Röntgenstr 1983 ;139:510-515.

86. **Grossman ZD**, Winstow BW, Bryan PJ, Dinn WM. Radionuclide imaging, computed tomography and gray-scale ultrasonography of the liver: a comparative study. J Nucl Med 1977; 18:327-332.

87. **Haggar AM**, Kressel HY. Magnetic resonance imaging of the genitourinary tract. Urol Clin N Am 1985; 12:725-736.

88. **Hahn EL.** Spin echoes. Phys Rev 1950; 80:580-594.

89. **Hahn FJ**, Wei-Kom Chu, Coleman PE et al. Artifacts and diagnostic pitfalls of magnetic resonance imaging: a clinical review. Rad Clin N Am 1988; 26:717-737.

90. **Hamlin DJ,** Cockett ATK. Computed tomography of bladder: staging of bladder cancer using low density opacification technique. Urology 1979; 13:331-334.

91. **Hamlin DJ,** Cockett ATK, Burgener FA. Computed tomography of the pelvis: sagittal and coronal image reconstruction in the evaluation of infiltrative bladder carcinoma. J Comp Ass Tom 1981; 5:27-33.

92. **Hansen G,** Crooks L, Davis P, et al. In vivo imaging of the rat anatomy with nuclear magnetic resonance. Radiology 1980; 136:695-700.

93. **Hawks RC,** Holland GN, Moore WS, Worthington BS. Nuclear magnetic resonance (NMR) tomography of the brain: a preliminary clinical assessment with demonstration of pathology. J Comp Ass Tom 1980; 4:577-586.

94. **Haynor DR,** Mack LA, Soules MR et al. Changing appearance of the normal uterus during the menstrual cycle: MR studies. Radiology 1986; 161:459-462.

95. **Heiken JP,** Lee JKT. MR imaging of the pelvis. Radiology 1988; 166:11-16.

96. **Hendee WR,** Morgan CJ. Magnetic resonance imaging: Part I. Physical principles. West J Med 1984; 141:491-495.

97. **Hendrick RE,** Nelson TR, Hendee WR. Optimizing tissue contrast in magnetic resonance imaging. Mag Res Im 1984; 2:193-204.

98. **Hendrick RE,** Newman FD, Hendee WR. Maximizing the signal to noise ratio from a single tissue. Radiology 1985; 156:749-752.

99. **Hendrick RE,** Osborn AG. Introduction to MR imaging. Part 2. Pulse sequences and image contrast. In: Syllabus: a categorical course in diagnostic radiology. MR imaging. Stark DD, Bradley WG, eds. 74th RSNA nov 27-dec 2, 1988:15-25.

100. **Hendrick RE.** Image contrast and noise. In: Magnetic resonance imaging Stark DD, Bradley WG, eds. 1988:66-83, St Louis, Mosby.

101. **Hendriks AJM,** Barentsz JO, Stappen WAH et al. The value of intravesical ultrasound combined with double surface coil MRI in staging bladder cancer. Brit Journ Urol 1989; 63:469-475.

102. **Hildell JG,** Nyman URO, Norlindh ST, et al. New intravesical contrast medium for CT: preliminary studies with arachis (peanut oil). AJR 1981; 137:777-780.

103. **Hillman BJ,** Silvert M, Cook G, et al. Recognition of bladder tumors by excretory urography. Radiology 1981; 138:319-323.

104. **Hinshaw WS,** Bottomley PA, Holland GN. Radiographic thin-section imaging of the human wrist by nuclear magnetic resonance. Nature 1977; 270:722-723.

105. **Hodson NJ,** Husband JE, Macdonald JS. The role of computed tomography in the staging of bladder cancer. Clin Radiology 1979; 30:389-395.

106. **Hricak H,** Williams RD, Spring DB, et al. Anatomy and pathology of the male pelvis by magnetic resonance imaging. AJR 1983; 141:1101-1110.

107. **Hricak H,** Alpers C, Crooks LE, Sheldon PE. Magnetic resonance imaging of the female pelvis: initial experience. AJR 1983; 141:1119-1128.

108. **Hricak H,** Crooks L, Sheldon P, Kaufman L. Nuclear magnetic resonance imaging of the kidney. Radiology 1983; 146:425-432.

109. **Hricak H.** MRI of female pelvis: review. AJR 1986; 146:1115-1122.

110. **Hricak H,** Chang YCF, Thurnher S. Vagina evaluation with MR imaging. Part I. Normal anatomy and congenital anomalies. Radiology 1988; 169:169-174.

111. **Hricak H,** Marotti M, Gilbert TJ et al. Normal penile anatomy and abnormal penile conditions: evaluation with MR imaging. Radiology 1988; 169:683-690.

112. **Hricak H,** Chang YCF. Female pelvis. In: Syllabus: a categorical course in diagnostic radiology. MR imaging. Stark DD, Bradley WG, eds. 74th RSNA meeting 1988:141-148.

113. **Inden Kleef J.** Interpolative interpretation of T_1- and T_2-relaxation times. Magnetic Resonance Imaging 1987; 5: 513-524.

114. **Itzack Y,** Singer D, Fischelovitch Y. Ultrasonographic assessment of bladder tumors. Tumor detection. J Urol 1981; 126:31-36.

115. **Jäger N,** Radeke HW, Adolphs HD, et al. Value of intravesical sonography in tumor clasification of bladder carcinoma. Eur Urol 1986; 12:76-84.

116. **Janetschek G,** Jaske G, Egeender G, zur Nedden D. Der Stellenwert der endovesicale Sonographie. Verh dt Ges Urol 1983; 35:221-222.

117. **Jeffry RB,** Palubinskas AJ, Federle MP. CT evaluation of invasive lesions of the bladder. J Comp Ass Tom 1981; 5:22-26.

118. **Jewett HJ,** Strong GH. Infiltrating carcinoma of the bladder. Relation of depth of penetration of the bladder wall to incidence of local extension and metastasis. J Urol 1946; 55:366-372.

119. **Jewett HJ.** Cancer of the bladder. Cancer 1973; 32:1072-1075.

120. **Johnson DE,** Kaesler KE, Kaminsky S, et al. Lymphangiography as an aid in staging bladder carcinoma. South Med J 1979; 69:28-30.

121. **Kademian MT,** Wirtanen GW. Accuracy of bipedal lympography in Hodgkin's disease. AJR 1977; 129:1041-1042.

122. **Katz JM,** Herman PG. Whole lung tomography in the oncology patient: indications and yield. Postgraduate Radiology 1981; 1.

123. **Kellet MJ,** Oliver RTD, Husband JE, Fry IK. Computed tomography as an adjunct to bimanual examination for staging bladder tumors. Br J Urol 1980; 52:101-106.

124. **Kenny GM,** Hardner GJ, Murphy GP. Clinical staging of bladder tumors. J Urol 1970; 104:720-723.

125. **Knight WD.** Nuclear magnetic shifts in metals. Phys Rev 1949; 76:1259-1260.

126. **Koebel G,** Schmeidl U, Griebel J et al. MR imaging of urinary bladder neoplasms. J Comp Ass Tom 1988; 12:98-103.

127. **König HA,** Laub G. Verarbetung und Darstellung dreidimensionaler Datensaetze in der Kernspintomographie. Electro Medica 1988; 2:42-50.

128. **Kools-Obdeyn IM,** Barentsz JO. Indicaties voor MRI in de obstetrie. Referaat KUN Radiologie 1987.

129. **Koops W.** MR compendium 1987. Philips MSD; Eindhoven 1987.

130. **Koss JC,** Arger PH, Coleman BG, et al. CT staging of bladder cancer. AJR 1981; 137:359-362.

131. **Küper K,** Koelbel G, Schmeidl U. Kernspintomographische Untersuchungen von Harnblasenkarzinomen bei 1.5 Tesla. Fortschr Röntgenstr 1986; 144:674-680.

132. **Kulkarni MV,** Patton JA, Price RR. MR imaging using specialised coils. AJR 1985; 147:373-378.

133. **Laakman RW,** Kaufman B, Han JS et al. MR imaging in patients with metallic implants. Radiology 1985; 157:711-714.

134. **Lackner K,** Brecht G, Janson R et al. Wertigkeit der Computertomographie bei der Stadieneinteilung primarer Lymphknotenneoplasien. Fortschr Röntgenstr 1980; 132:21-30.

135. **Lang EK.** The röntgenographic assessment of bladder tumors. Cancer 1969; 23:717-724.

136. **Lauffer RB.** Paramagnetic metal complexes as water proton relaxation agents for NMR imaging: theory and design. Chem. Rev. 1987; 87:901-927.

137. **Lauterbur PC.** Image formation by induced local interactions: examples employing nuclear magnetic resonance. Nature 1973; 242:190-191.

138. **Lee JKT,** Stanley RJ, Sagel SS, McClennan BL. Accuracy of CT in detecting intra-abdominal and pelvic lymph node metastases from pelvic cancers. AJR 1978; 131:675-681.

139. **Lee JKT,** Rholl KS. Review article. MRI of the bladder and prostate. AJR 1986; 147:732-736.

140. **Lemmens JAM,** Barentsz JO, Ruijs JHJ. Magnetic resonance imaging (MRI). Gamma 1987; 37:235-239.

141. **Lemmens JAM,** Horn JR van, Boer J den, et al. MR imaging of 22 Charnley-Müller total hip prosthesis. Fortschr Röntgenstr 1986; 145:311-315.

142. **Lenz M Von,** Bautz W, Deimling M, Küper K. Kernspintomographie des männlichen Beckens. Fortschr Röntgenstr 1985; 143:507-520.

143. **Lewis E.** Screening for diffuse and focal liver diseases: the case for hepatic sonography. J Clin Ultrasound 1984; 12:67-71.

144. **Liboff RL.** Neuromagnetic thresholds. J Theor Biol 1980; 83:427-432.

145. **Lin MS.** Measurement of spin lattice relaxation times in double spin echo imaging. Magn Res Med 1984; 1:361-369.

146. **Lin MS.** Interpolative computation of spin-lattice relaxation times from signal ratios. Mag Res Med 1985; 2:234-244.

147. **Lufkin RB,** Votruba J, Reicher M et al. Solenoid surface coils in magnetic resonance imaging. AJR 1986; 146:409-412.

148. **Mansfield P,** Maudsley AA. Medical imaging by NMR. Br J Radiol 1977; 50:188-194.

149. **Marchal G,** Coenen Y, Wilms G, Baert AL. The accuracy of CT-scan in the diagnosis of retroperitoneal metastasis of malignant testicular tumors. Fortschr Röntgenstr 1978; 128:746-753.

150. **Marglin S,** Castellino RA. Lymphographic accuracy in 631 consecutive, previously untreated cases of Hodgkin disease and non-Hodgkin lymphoma. Radiology 1981; 140:351-353.

151. **Margulis AR,** Higgins CB, Kaufman L, Crooks LE. Clinical magnetic resonance imaging. Univ Calif Print 1983; 50:188-194.

152. **Marshall VF.** The relation of the pre-operative estimate to pathologic demonstration of the extent of vesical neoplasms. J Urol 1952; 68:714-719.

153. **McCarthy S,** Tauber C, Gore J. Female pelvic anatomy: MR assessment of variations during the menstrual cycle and with use of oral contraceptives. Radiology 1986; 160:119-123.

154. **McNamara MT.** Monoclonal antibodies in magnetic resonance medical imaging. Sem Nucl Med 1983; 13:364-376.

155. **Meares EM.** Current problems in therapy of carcinoma of the bladder, testis and prostate. Urol Digest 1971; 19:13-18.

156. **Mechlin M,** Thickman D, Kressel HY et al. Magnetic resonance imaging of postoperative patients with metallic implants. AJR 1984; 143:1281-1285.

157. **Meijden van der APM.** Non specific immunotherapy with BCG-RIVM in superficial bladder cancer. Proefschrift 1988. Helmond, Wibro.

158. **Mills TC,** Ortendahl DA, Hylton NM et al. Partial flip angle MR imaging. Radiology 1987; 162:531-539.

159. **Moon KL,** Hricak H, Crooks LE et al. Nuclear magnetic resonance imaging of the adrenal gland: a preliminary report. Radiology 1983; 147:155-160.

160. **Moore BR.** Is the homing pigeon's map geomagnetic? Nature 1980; 285:69-75.

161. **Morgan CL,** Phil M, Calkins RF, Cavalcanti EJ. Computed tomography in the evaluation, staging and therapy of carcinoma of the bladder and prostate. Radiology 1981; 140:751-761.

162. **Morris PG.** Nuclear magnetic resonance imaging in medicine and body. Claredon Press, Oxford 1986.

163. **Murayama M.** Orientation of sickled erythrocytes in a magnetic field. Nature 1965; 202:420-424.

164. **Murphy GP.** Developments in preoperative staging of bladder tumors. Urology 1978; 11:109-115.

165. **National radiological protection board.** Revised guidance on acceptable limits of exposure during nuclear magnetic resonance clinical imaging. Br J Radiol 1983; 56:974-980.

166. **New PFJ,** Rosen BR, Brady TJ, et al. Potential hazards and artifacts of ferromagnetic and nonferromagnetic surgical and dental materials and devices in nuclear magnetic resonance imaging. Radiology 1985; 147:139-148.

167. **Nicolas V,** Harder T, Steudel A et al. Die Wertigkeit bildgebender Verfahren bei der Diagnostik und dem Stagierung von Harnblasentumoren. Fortschr Röntgenstr 1988; 148:234-239.

168. **Nunnally RL,** Bottomley PA. Assessment of pharmacological treatment of myocardial infarction by Phosphorus-31 NMR with surface coils. Science 1980; 211:177-180.

169. **Opella SJ.** Biological nuclear magnetic resonance spectroscopy. Science 1977; 198:158-165.

170. **Oppelt A,** Graumann R, Barfub H et al. FISP -a new fast MRI sequence. Electro Medica 1986; 54:15-18.

171. **Osborn AG,** Hendrick RE. Introduction to MR imaging. Part 1. Basic physics and instrumentation. In: Syllabus: a categorical course in diagnostic radiology. MR imaging. Stark DD, Bradley WG, eds. 74th RSNA meeting 1988:7-15.

172. **Paoletti PP,** Tenti S, Fiorelli C, et al. Lèchografia endocavitaria transuretrale. Urologia 1982; 49:648-654.

173. **Persson BRR.** Potential health hazards and safety aspects of clinical NMR examinations. Lasarettet, Lund 1984:178-181.

174. **Pfitzenmaier N,** Ikinger U, Möhring K. Transurethrale Sonographie -eine neue Methode zur Stadieneinteilung von Blasentumoren? N-Rhein Westf Ges Ur 1982:28-33.

175. **Phillips ME,** Kressel HY, Spritzer CE et al. Normal prostate and adjacent structures: MR imaging at 1.5 T. Radiology 1987; 164:381-385.

176. **Polga JP,** Watnick M. Whole lung tomography in metastatic disease. Clin Radiol 1976; 27:53-56.

177. **Prando A,** Wallace S, Von Eschenbach AC et al. Lymphangiography in the staging of carcinoma of the prostate. The potential value of percutaneous lymph node biopsy. Radiology 1979; 131:641-645.

178. **Proctor WG,** Yu FC. The dependence of a nuclear magnetic resonance frequency upon chemical compound. Phys Rev 1950; 77:717-723.

179. **Prout GR,** Slack NH, Bross IDJ. Preoperative irradiation as an adjuvant in the surgical management of invasive bladder carcinoma. J Urol 1971; 105:223-227.

180. **Purcell EM,** Torrey HC, Pound RV. Resonance absorption by nuclear magnetic moments in a solid. Phys Rev 1946; 70:460-474.

181. **Pusey E,** Lufkin RB, Brown RKJ et al. Magnetic resonance imaging artifacts: mechanism and clinical significance. Radiographics 1986; 6:891-911.

182. **Radda GK,** Seeley PJ. Recent studies on cellular metabolism by nuclear magnetic resonance. Ann Rev Physiol 1941; 41:749-753.

183. **Redman HC,** Glatstein E, Castellino RA, Federal WA. Computed tomography as an adjunct in the staging of Hodgkin's disease and non-Hodgkin's lymphomas. Radiology 1977; 124:381-385.

184. **Reiman TH,** Heiken JP, Totty WG, Lee JKT. Clinical MR imaging with a Helmholtz-type surface coil. Radiology 1988; 169:564-566.

185. **Renshaw PF,** Owen CS, Evans AE, Leigh JS. Immunospecific NMR contrast agents. Magn Res Im 1986; 4:351-357.

186. **Requardt H,** Sauter R, Weber H. Helmholtzspulen in der Kernspintomographie. Electromed 1987; 55:61-72.

187. **Resnick MI,** Kursh ED. Transurethral ultrasonography in bladder cancer. J Urol 1986; 135:253-255.

188. **Rholl KS,** Lee JKT, Heiken JP, et al. Primary bladder carcinoma: evaluation with MR imaging. Radiology 1987; 163:117-123.

189. **Richie JP,** Skinner DG, Kaufmann JJ. Carcinoma of the bladder: treatment by radical cystectomy. J Surg Res 1975; 18:271-277.

190. **Roy OZ.** Summary of cardiac fibrillation thresholds for 60 Hz currents and voltages applied directly to the heart. Med Biol Engineering & Comp 1980 :18-23.

191. **Rozsahegyi J von,** Magasi P, Goeblyoes P, et al. Der Wert der Ultrasonographie in der Harnblasentumordiagnostik. Fortschr Roentgenstr 1985; 143:431-437.

192. **Ruijs JHJ,** Koopmans JH. The costs of MR (MRI). A calculation for the Netherlands. Diagnostic Imaging 1986; 55:92-98.

193. **Runge VA,** Wood, ML, Kaufmann DM et al. FLASH: clinical three-dimensional magnetic resonance imaging. Radiographics 1988; 5:947-967.

194. **Runge VM,** Clanton JA, Lukehart CM et al. Paramagnetic agents for contrast enhanced NMR imaging: a review. AJR 1983; 141:1209-1215.

195. **Runge VM,** Schöner W, Niendorf et al. Initial clinical evaluation of gadolinium DTPA for contrast enhanced magnetic resonance imaging. Magn Res Imag 1985; 3:27-35.

196. **Runge VM,** Clanton JA, Price AC et al. The use of GD-DTPA as a perfusion agent and marker of blood-brain barrier disruption. Magn Res Imag 1985; 3:43-55.

197. **Sager EM,** Talle K, Fossa S, et al. The role of CT in demonstrating perivesical tumor growth in the preoperative staging of carcinoma of the urinary bladder. Radiology 1983; 146:443-446.

198. **Salo JO,** Kivisaari L, Lehtonen T. CT in determining the depth of infiltration of bladder tumors. Urol Radiology 1985; 7:88-93.

199. **Sauter R,** Requardt H, Weber H. Kernspintomographie mit anwendungsspezifisch entwickelten Hochfrequenzantennen. Electromed 1986; 54:96-101.

200. **Scher HI,** Yagoda A, Herr HW, et al. Neo-adjuvant M-VAC effect on the primary bladder lesion. J Urol 1987; 138:1402-1406.

201. **Schmidtbauer CP,** Schrameck P, Studler G. Stadieneinteilung von Primär Tumor und Rezidiv beim Blasenkarzinom durch endovesikale Sonographie. Verh dt Ges Urol 1983; 35:223-226.

202. **Schmidt JD,** Weinstein SH. Pitfalls in clinical staging of bladder tumors. Urol Clin N Am 1976; 3:107-127.

203. **Schüller J,** Walther V, Schmiedt E et al. Intravesical ultrasound tomography in staging bladder carcinoma. J Urol 1982; 128:264-266.

204. **Seidenwurm D,** Smathers RL, Lo RK et al. Testes and scrotum: MR imaging at 1.5.T. Radiology 1987; 164:393-398.

205. **Siedelmann FE,** Cohen WN, Bryan PJ. Computed tomographic staging of bladder neoplasms. Rad Clin N Am 1977; 15:419-440.

206. **Siedelmann FE,** Cohen WN, Bryan PJ et al. Accuracy of CT staging of bladder neoplasms using the gas-filled method: report of 21 patients with surgical conformation. AJR 1978; 130:735-739.

207. **Sigal R.** Magnetic resonance imaging: basis for interpretation. Springer Verlag 1988; 1st ed, Berlin, New York.

208. **Simeone JF,** Edelman RR, Stark DD. Surface coil MR imaging of the abdominal viscera. Part III. The pancreas. Radiology 1985; 157:437-441.

209. **Skinner DG,** Daniels JR, Lieskovsky G. Current status of adjuvant chemotherapy after radical cystectomy for deeply invasive bladder cancer. Urology 1984; 24:46-52.

210. **Soulen RL,** Budinger TF, Higgins CB. Magnetic resonance imaging of prosthetic heart valves. Radiology 1985; 154:705-707.

211. **Sternberg CN,** Yagoda A, Scher HI, et al. Preliminary results of M-VAC for transitional cell carcinoma of the urothelium. J Urol 1985; 133:403-407.

212. **Strijk SP,** Debruyne FMJ, Herman CJ. Lymphography in the management of urologic tumors. Radiology 1983; 146:39-45.

213. **Sullivan DL,** Taylor KJW, Gottschalk A. The use of ultrasound to enhance the diagnostic utility of the equivocal liver scintigraphy. Radiology 1978; 128:727-731.

214. **Trubowitz S,** Davis S. The bone marrow matrix. In: The human bone marrow: anatomy, pathology and pathophysiology. Boca Raton, Fla: CRC 1982:43-75.

215. **U.I.C.C.** TNM classification of malignant tumors. Ed.: Harmer MH; 3rd. ed. 1978, Geneva.

216. **U.I.C.C.** TNM classification of malignant tumors. Ed.: Harmer MH; 4th. ed. 1987, Geneva.

217. **Valk J,** MacLean C, Algra PR. Inleiding in de kernspintomografie (NMR imaging). VU Uitgeverij Amsterdam 1985, Amsterdam.

218. **Varkarakis MJ,** Gaeta J, Moore RH, et al. Superficial bladder tumors: aspects of clinical progression. Urology 1974; 4:414-419.

219. **Vavdin F,** Guiter J, Averous M et al. Apport de l'imagerie par resonance magnetique nucleaire (IRM) dans l'exploration urologique du pelvis masculin. Journ d'Urologie 1986; 8:509-520.

220. **Vock P,** Haertel M, Fuchs WA et al. Computed tomography in staging carcinoma of the urinary bladder. Br J Radiol 1982; 54:158-163.

221. **Vogler JB,** Murphy WA. Bone marrow imaging. Radiology 1988; 168:679-693.

222. **Walsh JW,** Amendola MA, Konerding KF, et al. Computed tomographic detection of pelvic and inguinal lymph node metastases from primary and recurrent pelvic malignant disease. Radiology 1980; 137:157-166.

223. **Wasjman Z,** Baumgarter G, Murphy GP, Merrin C. Evaluation of lymphangiography for clinical staging of bladder tumors. J Urol 1975; 114:712-714.

224. **Wasjman Z,** Merrin C, Moore R, Murphy GP. Current results from treatment of bladder tumors with total cystectomy at Roswell Park Memorial Institute. J Urol 1975; 113:806-810.

225. **Weinerman PM,** Arger PH, Pollack HM. CT evaluation of bladder and prostate neoplasms. Urol Radiology 1982; 4:105-114.

226. **Weisman ID,** Bennet LH. Recognition of cancer in vivo by nuclear magnetic resonance. Science 1972; 178:1288-1290.

227. **White EM,** Edelman RR, Strak DD. Surface coil MR imaging of the abdominal viscera. Part II. The adrenal gland. Radiology 1985; 157:431-436.

228. **Whitmore WF,** Batata MA, Ghoneim MA, Grabstald H, Unal A. Radical cystectomy with or without prior irradiation in the treatment of bladder cancer. J Urol 1977; 118:184-187.

229. **Winkler M,** Hricak H. Pelvis imaging with MR: technique for improvement. Radiology 1986; 158:848-849.

230. **Wolf GL,** Joseph PM en Goldstein EJ. Optimal pulsing sequences for MR contrast agents. AJR 1986; 147:367-371.

231. **Wolff S,** Crooks LE, Brown P et al. Tests for DNA and chromosomal damage induced by NMR imaging. Radiology 1980; 136:707-710.

232. **Wolff S.** Magnetic resonance imaging: absence of in vitro cytogenetic damage. Radiology 1985; 155:163-165.

233. **Yagoda A.** Progress in chemotherapy for cancers of the urothelium. Urology 1984; 23:118-123.

234. **Yu WS,** Sagerman RH, King GA, et al, The value of computed tomography in the management of bladder cancer. Int J Radiat Oncol Biol Phys 1979; 5:135-142.

235. **Ziedes des Plantes Jr BG.** Potential hazards of magnetic resonance imaging. In: Essentials of clinical MRI. Falke THM (ed). Martinus Nijhof Publ. 1988:17-24. Dordrecht, Boston, Lancaster.

SERIES IN RADIOLOGY

1. J. O. Op den Orth: *The Standard Biphasic-contrast Examination of the Stomach and Duodenum.* Method, Results, and Radiological Atlas. 1979   ISBN 90–247–2159–8
2. J. L. Sellink and R. E. Miller: *Radiology of the Small Bowel.* Modern Enteroclysis Technique and Atlas. 1982   ISBN 90–247–2460–0
3. R. E. Miller and J. Skucas: *The Radiological Examination of the Colon.* Practical Diagnosis. 1983   ISBN 90–247–2666–2
4. S. Forgács: *Bones and Joints in Diabetes Mellitus.* 1982   ISBN 90–247–2395–7
5. Gy. Németh and H. Kuttig (eds.): *Isodose Atlas for Use in Radiotherapy.* 1981   ISBN 90–247–2476–7
6. J. Chermet: *Atlas of Phlebography of the Lower Limbs.* Including the Iliac Veins. 1982   ISBN 90–247–2525–9
7. B. K. Janevski: *Angiography of the Upper Extremity.* 1982   ISBN 90–247–2684–0
8. M. A. M. Feldberg: *Computed Tomography of the Retroperitoneum.* An Anatomical and Pathological Atlas with Emphasis on the Fascial Planes. 1983   ISBN 0–89838–573–3
9. L. E. H. Lampmann, S. A. Duursma and J. H. J. Ruys: *CT Densitometry in Osteoporosis.* The Impact on Management of the Patient. 1984   ISBN 0–89838–633–0
10. J. J. Broerse and T. J. Macvittie: *Response of Different Species to Total Body Irradiation.* 1984   ISBN 0–89838–678–0
11. C. L'Herminé: *Radiology of Liver Circulation.* 1985   ISBN 0–89838–715–9
12. G. Maatman: *High-resolution Computed Tomography of the Paranasal Sinuses, Pharynx and Related Regions.* Impact of CT Identification on Diagnosis and Patient Management. 1986   ISBN 0–89838–802–3
13. C. Plets, A. L. Baert, G. L. Nijs and G. Wilms: *Computer Tomographic Imaging and Anatomic Correlation of the Human Brain.* A Comparative Atlas of Thin CT-scan Sections and Correlated Neuro-anatomic Preparations. 1987   ISBN 0–89838–811–2
14. J. Valk: *MRI of the Brain, Head, Neck and Spine.* A Teaching Atlas of Clinical Applications. 1987   ISBN 0–89838–957–7
15. J. L. Sellink: *X-Ray Differential Diagnosis in Small Bowel Disease.* A Practical Approach. 1988   ISBN 0–89838–351–X
16. Th.H.M. Falke (ed.): *Essentials of Clinical MRI.* 1988   ISBN 0–89838–353–6
17. B. D. Fornage: *Endosonography.* 1989   ISBN 0–7923–0047–5
18. R. Chisin (ed.): *MRI/CT and Pathology in Head and Neck Tumors.* A Correlative Study. 1989   ISBN 0–7923–0227–3
19. G. Gozzetti, A. Mazziotti, L. Bolondi and L. Barbara (eds.): *Intraoperative Ultrasonography in Hepato-biliary and Pancreatic Surgery.* A Practical Guide. With Contributions by Y. Chapuis, J.-F. Gigot and P.-J. Kestens. 1989   ISBN 0–7923–0261–3
20. A. M. A. De Schepper and H. R. M. Degryse: *Magnetic Resonance Imaging of Bone and Soft Tissue Tumors and Their Mimics.* A Clinical Atlas. With Contributions by F. De Belder, L. van den Houwe, F. Ramon, P. Parizel and N. Buyssens. 1989   ISBN 0–7923–0343–1